## A PLACE IN MIND

**Commissioning and Providing Mental Health Services for People who are Homeless**

## EDITORS

Dr Richard Williams

and

Ms Kina Avebury

## AUTHORS

Ms Kina Avebury

Dr Simon Baugh

Ms Sarah Gorton

Mr David Laws

Mrs Dorothy Lott

Mr Ted Riley

Mr Mike Rodger

Professor Janine Scott

Dr Richard Williams

## PROJECT MANAGERS

Ms Kina Avebury

Mr Roderick Montgomery

# CHAPTER 1

Director's Introduction

*"Home is the place where, when you have to go there,
they have to take you in".*

*The Death of the Hired Man*
*Robert Frost*

1  The plight of homeless people in general, and homeless mentally ill people
in particular, has become an issue of increasing concern in the last decade.
From the point of view of the health services, this thematic review has
taught us that a group of people can clearly be seen as a barometer of
confidence in the service and the quality of care for two key reasons.

- First, the emphasis of mental health services has swung towards
community-based provision. There is a popular perception that
homeless mentally ill people are exemplars of the failure of the policy
of community care. While this idea may be inaccurate, improvement
in the standard of services and the co-ordination between hospital
and community teams is needed to ensure public confidence in this
approach.

- Second, homeless mentally ill people are at the extreme end of the
broad spectrum of disadvantage. Often, they are multiply deprived
and present health and social services with more complex problems
to resolve than people who are satisfactorily housed. If services are
able to meet the needs of homeless mentally ill people, they are likely
to be able to respond appropriately to most other groups in the
community.

2  Thus, the development of effective and accessible mental health services
for homeless people presents an opportunity not only to provide services
to a vulnerable group in the community, but also to improve the standards
of mental health services generally.

3  While most mental health services treat considerable numbers of
homeless people, many professionals remain unaware of the different
sub-groups within the homeless population, and the nature and extent of
their mental health problems and their differing service needs. It is
disappointing to note that, nationally, only 6% of health authorities
specifically mentioned homelessness as an issue in the service specifications
drawn up between purchasers and providers for 1993-4.

## THE INTENTIONS OF THIS REVIEW

4  The aim of this thematic review is to offer information and guidance on the
commissioning and provision of mental health services to people who are
homeless. While the review is addressed mainly to NHS managers, much of
the material relates to the social services and housing departments of local
authorities. The main thrust of this report is on joint working. The authors of
the review are aware that homelessness on its own, or in association with
mental health problems, is not always recognised as a major issue by health
and social services managers, and that the particular needs of a highly
vulnerable group of people may, therefore, remain unmet. This report
examines the characteristics of the homeless population and identifies the
specific challenges that it presents both to managers, in their development
of strategy for commissioning, and to front-line providers of services. This
report identifies examples of good practice across England and Wales.

5   The review was built on three foundations. First, it contains an appraisal of the existing literature on homelessness and mental illness in England and Wales, with some comparative references to studies of the North American picture. Second, it builds upon the programme of service visits undertaken by the NHS Health Advisory Service to 10 locations in England and Wales and, third, it incorporates the views and experiences of people who have first-hand knowledge of what it means to be homeless and mentally ill.

## RECENT POLICY CHANGES

6   This report makes reference to recent policy initiatives as well as to recent and proposed changes in legislation. These include:

*The Patients' Charter*
*The NHS and Community Care Act 1990*
*The Health of the Nation strategic initiative launched in England in 1992*
*Mental Illness - A Strategy for Wales launched in 1989*
*The Welsh Office NHS Directorate's Protocol for Investment in Health Gain - Mental Health (dated 1993)*
*Proposals for Supervised Discharge and Supervision Registers*
*The Criminal Justice and Public Order Act 1994*
*Proposed Changes to the Housing Act 1985*

7   These measures are examined in the context of homelessness and their likely impact upon homeless mentally ill people.

## THE CURRENT SITUATION

8   The survey of the literature provided in this text summarises some basic facts and figures on the incidence of homelessness. There is general agreement that it is rising significantly, and that the figures doubled between 1980 and 1990. The mean age of the homeless population is falling steadily and the gender distribution is changing, with the rate of increase in the number of homeless women (with and without children) outstripping that of men.

9   Government statistics record that, in 1992, local authorities accepted 148,250 households as homeless, a threefold increase since 1978. These figures represent one third of the number of people who applied for accommodation as homeless in that year under the provision of the Housing Act 1985.

10   The review found that, overall, inner London still has the highest prevalence of registered homelessness with 4.0 per 1,000 households against 1.6 per 1,000 households for the rest of England. However, the review also found that, while London is seen as the most problematic area in terms of homelessness, about two-thirds of homeless people live outside the capital. The rate of increase in the last decade has been 50% greater outside London, both in metropolitan and non-metropolitan districts. The greatest proportional increases were in the Midlands, Humberside and Yorkshire. This report also explores the issue of homelessness in rural areas and concludes that the position in these areas has developed with about 12% of the homeless population located in the country in or around market towns and villages. The likelihood of this group of people receiving services as a matter of priority is considered to be less than that of their urban counterparts.

11  Our review examined homelessness in a way which reflects a wide range of circumstances. It covers street homeless people, squatters, refugees, travellers, hostel and bedsitter residents, discharged psychiatric patients and people sleeping on friends' floors. It deals primarily, but not exclusively, with single homeless people and draws attention to the plight of hidden homeless people.

## THE METHODOLOGY

12  Members of the review team have assembled and examined the relevant studies on homelessness and its links with mental ill health undertaken in Britain and the United States over the past 20 years. This is presented together with a summary of recent changes in legislation and new Government policy initiatives and is followed by some general principles which have emerged in the course of the review on the provision of services for homeless people.

13  The initial exploratory work was followed by a programme of fieldwork visits to ten locations in England and Wales. The HAS teams met commissioners and providers of mental health services as well as voluntary agencies and housing and social services officers in local authorities. They also met some people who were currently using the mental health services. A distinctive feature of the review is the parallel programme of visits made by people who have experienced mental health problems themselves to service users in the same areas as those visited by the HAS teams. The detailed reports of all these visits have been synthesised into this review.

## ACKNOWLEDGEMENTS

### The Services

14  I would like to thank the staff of the many services interviewed in the course of the fieldwork. They gave freely of their time and knowledge. I hope that they recognise the aspects of good practice, drawn from their contributions, in this document and that this report makes them feel their efforts were worthwhile.

### The Authors

15  My special thanks are due to the authors of this document (Annex A). They have led the preparation of this report with dedication and attention to detail and responded positively to requests for information and fresh drafts, often at short notice.

### The Steering Committee and Service Visitors

16  I cannot thank all of these people sufficiently for their dedication to the task, time and support to me. Their biographies appear in Annexes A, B and C. Many of the members of the steering committee have undertaken tasks of considerable importance in drafting the initial documents on which the review of the literature and the fieldwork were based. Their experience, wisdom and dedication have formed the backbone of consistency throughout this review. They also spearheaded the service visits. Within that team, Kina Avebury has played a crucial role in providing consistency and practical strength throughout the project, in undertaking a number of the service visits, and in the drafting of this report.

17   Each member of this team of authors, steering committee members and service visitors has ensured that the thematic review has been guided with an appropriately broad perspective and one that acknowledges and draws on the contributions made by a wide range of professional disciplines in promoting the mental health of homeless people. They have responded to my deadlines yet ensured that considerable thought and wisdom has informed their work and I trust this document reflects some of their attention and sagacity.

**Dr Richard Williams**
**Director**
**NHS Health Advisory Service**

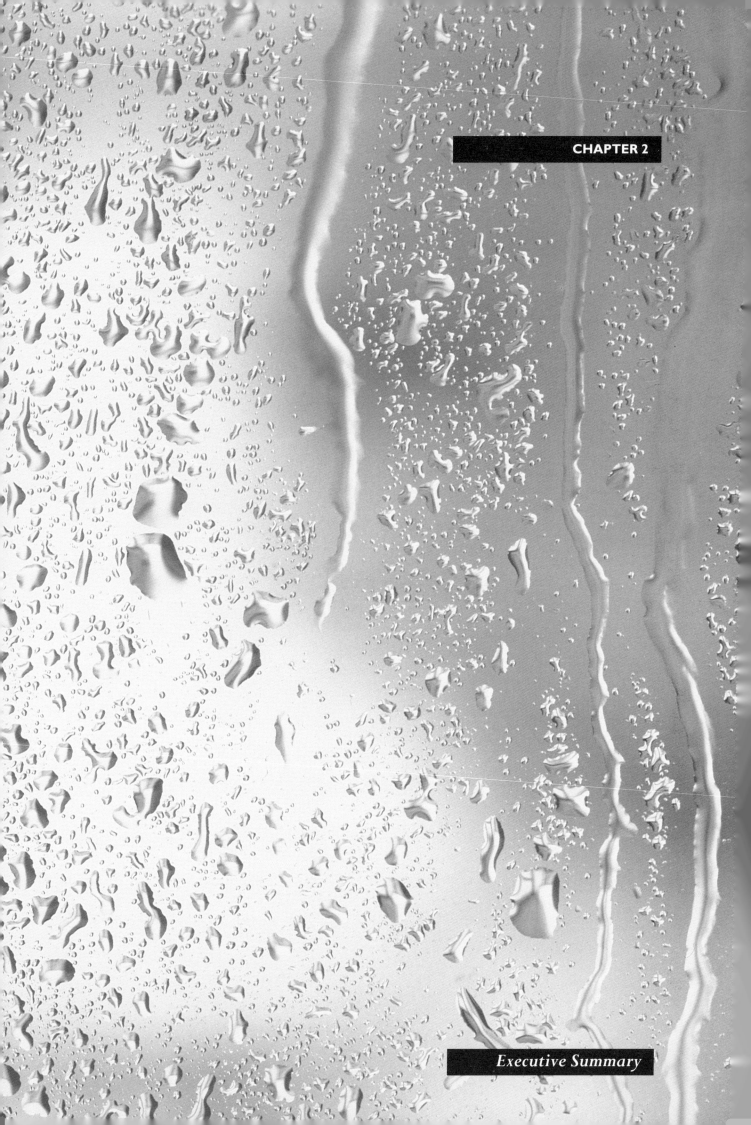

# CHAPTER 2

*Executive Summary*

18     This thematic review is concerned with homeless mentally ill people and how well they are served within the current structure of mental health services in England and Wales. The review has been carried out by a multi-disciplinary team, assembled by the NHS Health Advisory Service (HAS). This team comprised senior clinicians, health service managers, academics, local authority officers, the staff of voluntary sector organisations and others with considerable experience of mental health care for this particularly disadvantaged group. Team members have researched what is known about homeless mentally ill people, including definitions of homelessness, demographic distribution, social characteristics, clinical needs, approaches to provision and user perceptions about what is available to them. Team members also took part in a series of service visits, focused on provision for this client group, to commissioners and providers throughout England and Wales.

19     In this report, we aim to provide an understanding of the difficulties and challenges faced by mental health service clinicians and managers, in ensuring that homeless mentally ill people receive effective and appropriate care. We have not pulled any punches in presenting our findings, which represent a call for action, but we do highlight the many instances of good practice encountered in the research and field visits. These examples reinforce the importance of cross-agency working, the pooling of knowledge between voluntary and statutory sectors and provision that is properly monitored against specific service targets.

20     A significant part of the HAS teams' understanding has been derived from listening to service users; hearing what they say about their needs and experiences. Quotations from service users are placed throughout the text as a deliberate attempt to balance the sometimes conflicting views of those involved in the commissioning and providing sides of the discussion. In chapter eight, service users' accounts are presented in more detail.

## THE FINDINGS OF THE REVIEW

21     As a preliminary note to the findings that follow, it should be stated that the provision of care, be it mainstream health care or mental health care, for homeless people, is fraught with difficulties. The very nature of homelessness, involving a vicious circle of deprivation and marginalisation from the community, means that it is extremely difficult to locate and provide help for homeless individuals satisfactorily. A significant sector of this client group, as demonstrated by many of the quotes from users themselves and the user visitor reports, are deeply suspicious of statutory sector authorities of all kinds. While the prevailing support and care mechanisms for homeless mentally ill people are far from satisfactory and the various interfaces between this group and health care in its widest sense must be improved, there are manifold obstacles to effective provision, stemming from the fact that so many homeless people are 'hidden' or hide themselves from appropriate support and treatment.

22     We summarise the findings of the review as follows:

   -   It is estimated that there are between one and two million homeless people in Great Britain and they are distributed throughout England and Wales in rural as well as inner city areas. In the definition of homelessness adopted by reviewers in this report, we include people who literally have nowhere to live, as well as members of families who would normally live together but who live separately because they have nowhere to live together; and others whose accommodation is moveable (for example, travellers). This is not an exhaustive list but reveals a picture of a significant 'hidden' group of homeless people, which is why it is virtually impossible to give more than a broad figure for their numbers.

- The mean age of the homeless population is falling and the rate of increase of women (with and without children) is outstripping that of men.

- With the exception of a few inner city areas, homelessness is not perceived as a major concern. This is sometimes due to denial and sometimes to lack of relevant information, both about local sources of data and about the nature and size of the local homeless population.

- There is a high prevalence of mental health problems - including for example, enduring serious mental illness, alcohol and drug-related problems, personality disorders and chronic stress - among people who are homeless. There is also a significantly enhanced risk of suicide and deliberate self-harm in this client group.

- The voluntary sector is often the major provider of services to this client group. As such, it possesses knowledge, resources and skills in working with homeless people.

- Commissioning processes in the statutory sector seldom take account of the needs of homeless mentally ill people. Few strategy documents mention this group, while the knowledge-base for developing a comprehensive strategy is generally lacking.

- Few authorities have developed specially designated services for homeless people. Where these have been set up they have proved to be most effective, particularly where there is an explicit policy of working towards full integration with mainstream services.

- There are problems of getting homeless people registered with GPs. The situation is slightly easier in inner city areas. We examine the reasons for the difficulties for providing primary health care to homeless people in this review.

- There is considerable variation in the degree to which homeless people are the subjects of individual care planning (arising from the requirements of the Care Programme Approach and Section 117 of the Mental Health Act, 1983).

- The presence of a large number of 'travellers', both New Age and traditional, is a noticeable feature in Wales and the West of England. There are particular problems generated by seasonal migrations and a highly mobile population in general.

- There is a serious lack of effective co-operation between health purchasers and providers and housing services at planning and operational level.

## SEEKING LONG-TERM IMPROVEMENTS

23  These findings lead, in the review, to a closer examination of the challenges presented to those responsible for commissioning and purchasing mental health services. We place particular emphasis on the development of

strategies for commissioning mental health care for homeless people and on the importance of a sound knowledge-base. We also consider the roles of provider managers and clinicians, and the specific implications for their services as they attempt to respond to the needs of a vulnerable and marginalised group of people. Key elements affecting the provision of services for homeless people include the need for mature relationships between purchasers and providers, for healthy alliances with other stakeholders and for a willingness to consult and listen to local people, including service users.

24  We give particular emphasis to the concepts of working across agency boundaries, so that, for example, there is good liaison and joint strategy planning and other cross-agency communications within and between health services (purchasers and provider units; primary and secondary care; and community and hospital-based specialist care), social services and housing departments. We include recommendations on appropriate commissioning and purchasing practice and, in particular, on devising contracts which recognise the attributes and challenges of each area's particular homeless population. The contracting approach we propose addresses a wide range of issues and involves clearly agreed standards of care that can be monitored as part of a long-term process of service development. We also emphasise the importance of forming healthy alliances with the voluntary sector. These factors emerge as keys to providing effective mental health care for homeless people. The pooling of information, skills and resources offers the best way of meeting the challenges presented by this population.

25  To prepare the ground for much-needed improvements to mental health care for homeless mentally ill people, we have identified services, or elements of services, that demonstrate an effective approach to purchasing and provision for this group. In every area visited, the review teams noticed 'instances' where commendably high quality services were available, or where sensitivity to people with complex and challenging needs was clearly demonstrated. We illustrate these examples of good practice in the review. They are identified by area, with key learning points, and we hope they will stimulate authorities all over the country to explore possibilities for improvements to services in their own districts. The review concludes with a summary chapter presenting key concepts, that apply specifically to homeless mentally ill people, with corresponding challenges which these concepts present to managers, clinicians and commissioners.

26  While the current state of provision is generally in the range from poor to lamentable (with some noteworthy exceptions) there are a number of approaches that will ensure improvements. Briefly, examples include:

- Taking good note of specialist (often voluntary) services, which offer excellent examples of good practice as well as a source of skill and expertise and adapting such models to meet other, equally challenging needs.

- Improving access to all services - primary, secondary and long-term - for homeless people; this will help to reduce repeated hospital admissions and inappropriate contact with the prison system and health emergency services.

- Not least, the provision of housing, linked with carefully assessed clinical and social support, will move vulnerable homeless people away from the margins of existence, offering the chance of rehabilitation, recovery and re-entry into the community.

27    We envisage considerable benefits from the adoption of the approaches suggested in this review. A model where agencies plan and work together is likely to produce seamless and therefore more acceptable packages of care to people with multiple and complex needs.

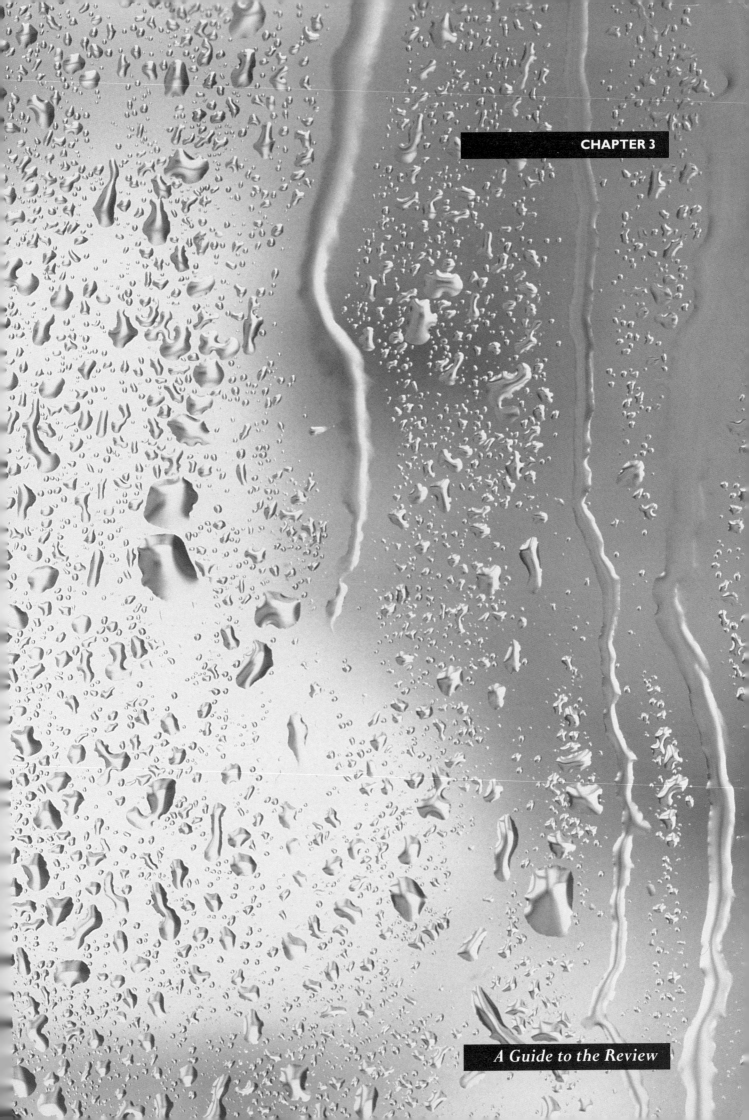

**CHAPTER 3**

*A Guide to the Review*

## AIM

28    This review aims to raise awareness of the mental health and associated problems faced by the homeless population and the potential service solutions that may be developed.

## THE CONTENTS OF THIS DOCUMENT

29    The introductory chapters describe why and how the thematic review was conducted.

30    Part A identifies important background data about homeless people, including the types of mental health and other problems encountered by this group of people. While highlighting the difficulties of gaining accurate information on the numbers of homeless people, this section also emphasises the need for service purchasers and providers to understand that homelessness is more than just rootlessness. People in temporary housing, and a variety of other settings, make up a hidden homeless population which also requires effective and accessible services.

31    The nature and extent of mental illness among the different homeless populations is documented and information is provided on possible pathways to homelessness. It will be apparent that the interplay between homelessness and mental illness is complex. Did homelessness arise in an individual as a consequence of mental illness (through inability to maintain work and housing; or as a consequence of poor discharge support following hospitalisation)? Did homelessness cause or lead to a worsening of mental illness in the individual (the stress of homelessness might precipitate a breakdown; or an individual with a mental illness who becomes homeless may then fail to receive appropriate follow-up treatment, such as medication, and then relapse)? All these individuals come under the umbrella of the population of homeless mentally ill people. Given the complexity of their problems, it is predictable that it is unlikely that there is a single service solution to meeting the needs of homeless mentally ill people.

32    Part A also presents the views of homeless people on current mental health services.

33    Part B (chapter nine) acknowledges the need to develop locally appropriate services. It outlines key principles that should ensure that homeless mentally ill people receive high quality services.

34    As such, the principles can be seen to systematise good clinical practice in specialist and mainstream services. They also highlight the impact of negative attitudes towards homeless people which, if not acknowledged and explored, may adversely influence the quality of care received by this very disadvantaged group of mentally ill people.

35    Part C of this report looks specifically at the issues confronting those who are commissioners. It covers the pre-requisites for determining effective strategy and the implications for commissioning and purchasing services for homeless people, in particular. This section also deals with the importance for commissioners of developing good working relationships with all stakeholders, including commissioners from other sectors of care, providers, local people, the voluntary sector, and service users.

A GUIDE TO THE REVIEW

*"I don't ever expect to be truly happy, but maybe life could be a little better than it is."*

*Quote from user*

36  Part C also offers guidance on the processes of commissioning services for homeless people. The stepping stones to good purchasing and the imperatives for effective contracting for this patient group, which have been built on the approach espoused by *Purchasing for Health*, are set out together with examples of good practice.

37  Part D switches the emphasis towards the providers of services. It offers guidance on the clinical tasks involved and the implications for provider managers. It also provides a number of examples of good practice in service provision, largely drawn from the experiences of the HAS teams which performed the visits to services.

38  Part E summarises the key concepts and challenges which have emerged during this review and provides checklists drawn from the text.

39  It must be emphasised again that we are providing potential rather than prescriptive solutions. The goal of this work is to share the considerable knowledge and expertise gained through the process of conducting the review to help others to provide high quality services to a disadvantaged and often stigmatised group.

## USING THE REVIEW

40  This review is written with a broad readership in mind. Every effort has been made to make it accessible by adding bullet points and tables. The background data in Parts A and B is intended to be read by everyone - there are many misconceptions regarding the identification and characteristics of people who could be described as being homeless and mentally ill. Common stereotypes bear little relationship to reality and to the facts concerning the spectrum of people to which this review draws attention.

41  While Part C, based on the format provided by *Purchasing for Health*, will be of particular interest to those involved in commissioning services, homeless people face multiple problems and many others from statutory and non-statutory provider agencies will clearly find that section of the document useful.

42  The chapter which offers *A Summary of Key Concepts and Challenges*, towards the end, draws together significant matters from all the earlier chapters and offers a summary of opinion on the elements underlying an effective local strategy for providing and monitoring effective services for homeless mentally ill people.

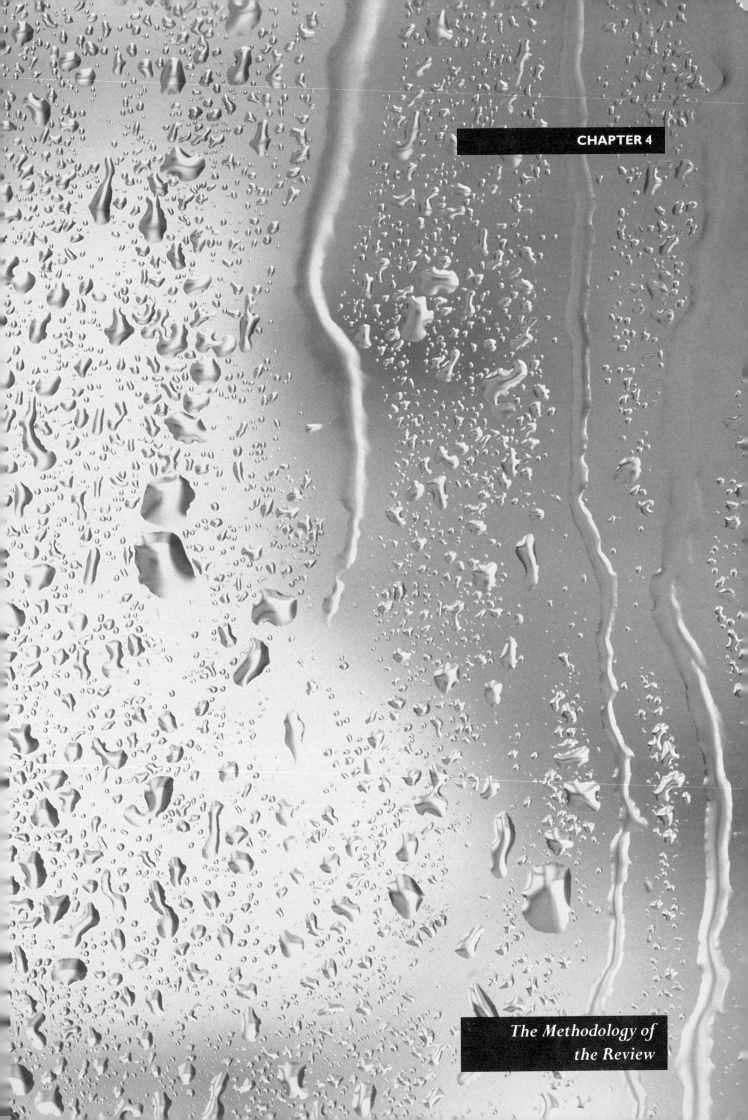

CHAPTER 4

*The Methodology of
the Review*

## THE BACKGROUND

THE METHODOLOGY OF
THE REVIEW

**43**    This thematic review has been guided by a steering committee which was set up in September 1992 to advise the Director of the NHS Health Advisory Service (HAS).

**44**    The membership of the steering committee (see Annexes A and B) was drawn widely from a range of people with varied professional backgrounds. These included academics, senior NHS managers from commissioning and providing organisations, leading-edge managers and professional staff from the health service, local authorities and the voluntary sector as well as general practitioners. All the members have had experience either of working directly with homeless mentally ill people or of research or of commissioning services for this client group.

**45**    The methodology is summarised in Figure 1.

*Figure 1*

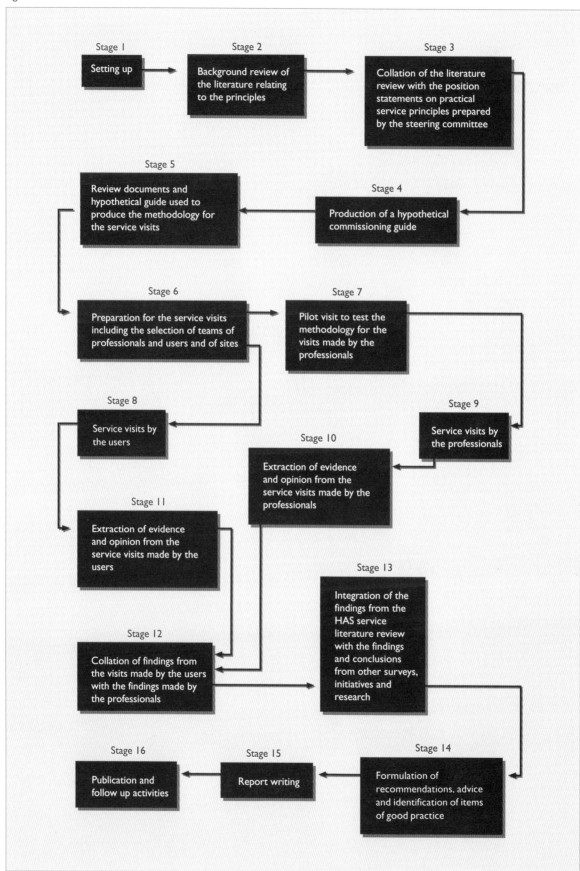

**46**  The early part of the work demanded a review of existing literature on the needs of homeless mentally ill people, and the differing responses to these needs in England and Wales and the United States of America. This led to the generation of a hypothetical document on commissioning mental health services for homeless people. This was subsequently used to create the methodology and questionnaires used in the service visits. The fieldwork visits to local services were then planned. Sub-groups of the steering committee met throughout 1993 to: draw up background documents; plan in greater detail; identify the key areas of concern; and draw up the checklists and questionnaires for the service visits. The service visits began in December 1993 with a pilot visit to a London Borough to test the methodology.

## THE SERVICE VISITS

**47**  Ten locations in England and Wales were identified as appropriate areas for service visits. They were chosen to achieve a representative spread of areas with differing characteristics rather than concentrating on those areas known to have large numbers of homeless people. The sample, therefore, covered: inner city, suburban and rural areas; seaside resorts; northern and southern sites. Eight of the locations visited were in England, and two were in Wales. The pilot visit was used to test the effectiveness of the pre-visit arrangements, the semi-structured questionnaires and the template for the processes of the visiting programme itself. Generally, all were considered to be satisfactory.

**48**  Each visit by teams (see Annexes A, B and C) on behalf of the HAS followed a similar pattern. Once agreement, relating to the dates and the broad outline of the fieldwork, was reached with the key senior managers of both health and social services purchasing authorities and their providers, questionnaires were mailed to a wide range of individuals and agencies in the area to be visited. These were targeted at particular departments or areas of responsibility and, while all the questionnaires were designed to elicit information on the provision of mental health services for homeless people, the questions were specific to the respondents.

**49**  Questionnaires were sent to:

- Directors of purchasing and contracts managers in health authorities and family health service authorities.

- Directors of social services and their staffs.

- General practitioners, both fundholding and non-fundholding.

- Health visitors.

- A range of mental health service personnel.

- Professional teams offering specialist mental health services, including crisis intervention, resettlement and drug and alcohol misuse services.

- Accident and emergency departments.

- Residential and day care project managers.

- Voluntary agencies working in the fields of homelessness and mental illness.

50    The completed questionnaires proved useful in many ways. They provided positive information on what services were available to homeless people, and on the operational links between services. They also demonstrated the real problems confronting purchasers and providers, who generally lacked information on the numbers and whereabouts of homeless people. General practitioners, in particular, showed a low level of awareness about the issues relating to homeless mentally ill people, and with very few exceptions, their responses indicated the absence of this group of people from their registers. Overall, these questionnaires were useful in equipping the HAS teams with information in advance of the visits and this was used as a basis for subsequent discussion during the interviews and meetings which made up the fieldwork programmes.

51    Each visit took place over three days. The opening meeting with senior officers of the health authorities set the scene. Other meetings took place with: senior social services officers; provider managers from trusts and directly managed units; general practitioners; staff of accident and emergency units; staff of acute medical and psychiatric inpatient services; professionals and managers from specialist teams, day centres, drop-in facilities, local authority homeless persons' units and hostels; voluntary sector staff and their clients; and also with officers of community health councils.

52    The programme of visits and meetings was intensive. It enabled a clear impression of the situation in each area to be gained quickly. After the pilot visit, the sequence of meetings was rearranged to allow discussion with the voluntary sector agencies to take place earlier in the three-day programme. This was because the teams realised how useful these agencies were in providing information on the extent of homelessness and of the particular problems of gaining access to services experienced by the people they were working with.

## THE OPINIONS OF SERVICE USERS

53    The visiting teams had limited opportunities to speak directly with homeless people who had mental health problems. This, on its own, was not considered to be a sufficiently effective way of getting a comprehensive view of what service users really felt about their needs and problems. The HAS attached great importance to finding out what the users' own perceptions were. Therefore, arrangements were made for the same 10 locations to be visited by people who have had direct experience of mental illness, and, sometimes, of homelessness. These 'user interviewers' were provided with lists of places where homeless mentally ill people might be found, for example night shelters, soup kitchens, day centres and direct access hostels. They were also provided with guidelines for interviews with service users.

54    The user interviewers produced extensive reports on their visits. These have, predictably, contained uncomfortable reading. Many homeless people expressed disillusion or active hostility towards the mental health 'system'. Some people felt that the most acceptable forms of support came not from statutory service providers, but from café owners, churches and self-help networks. The users' reports add weight to existing knowledge about the problems of access to services.

55 The authors of this report have made every effort to see that the users' perspectives have been integrated into the guidance which it now offers to commissioners and providers. They believe that the parallel exercise of user-to-user interviews alongside the more formal visits by managers and professionals has provided a sensitive way of seeking information which will be a useful baseline in offering improved services.

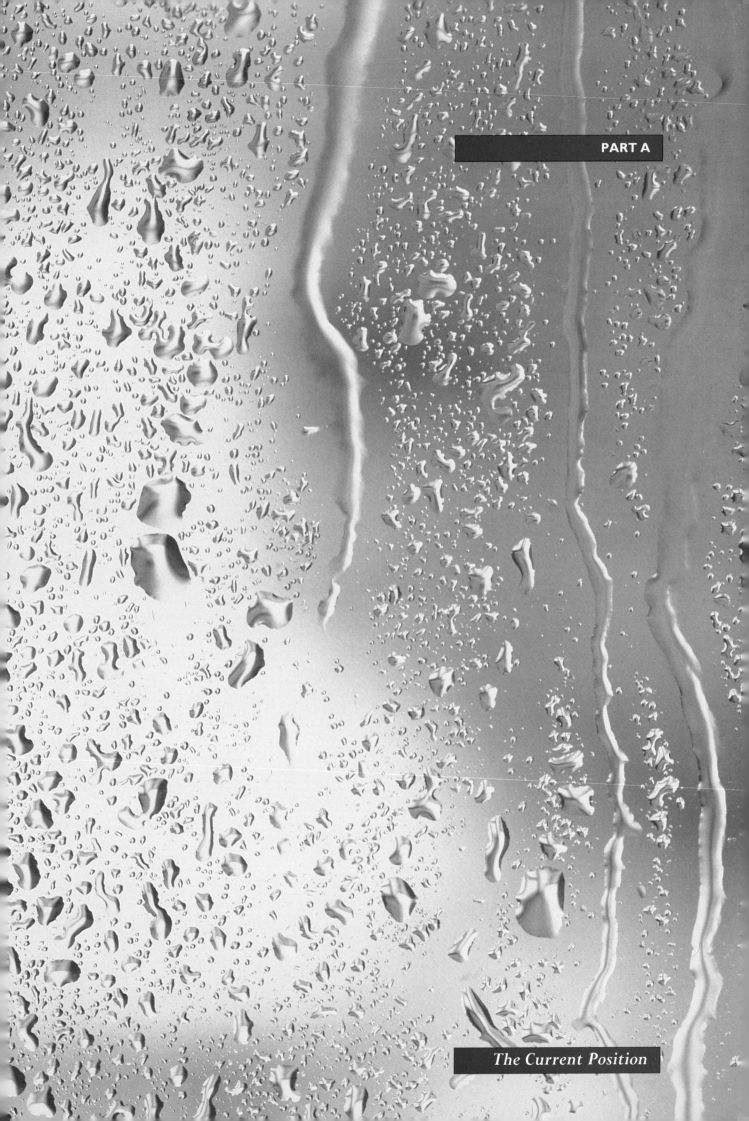

*The Current Position*

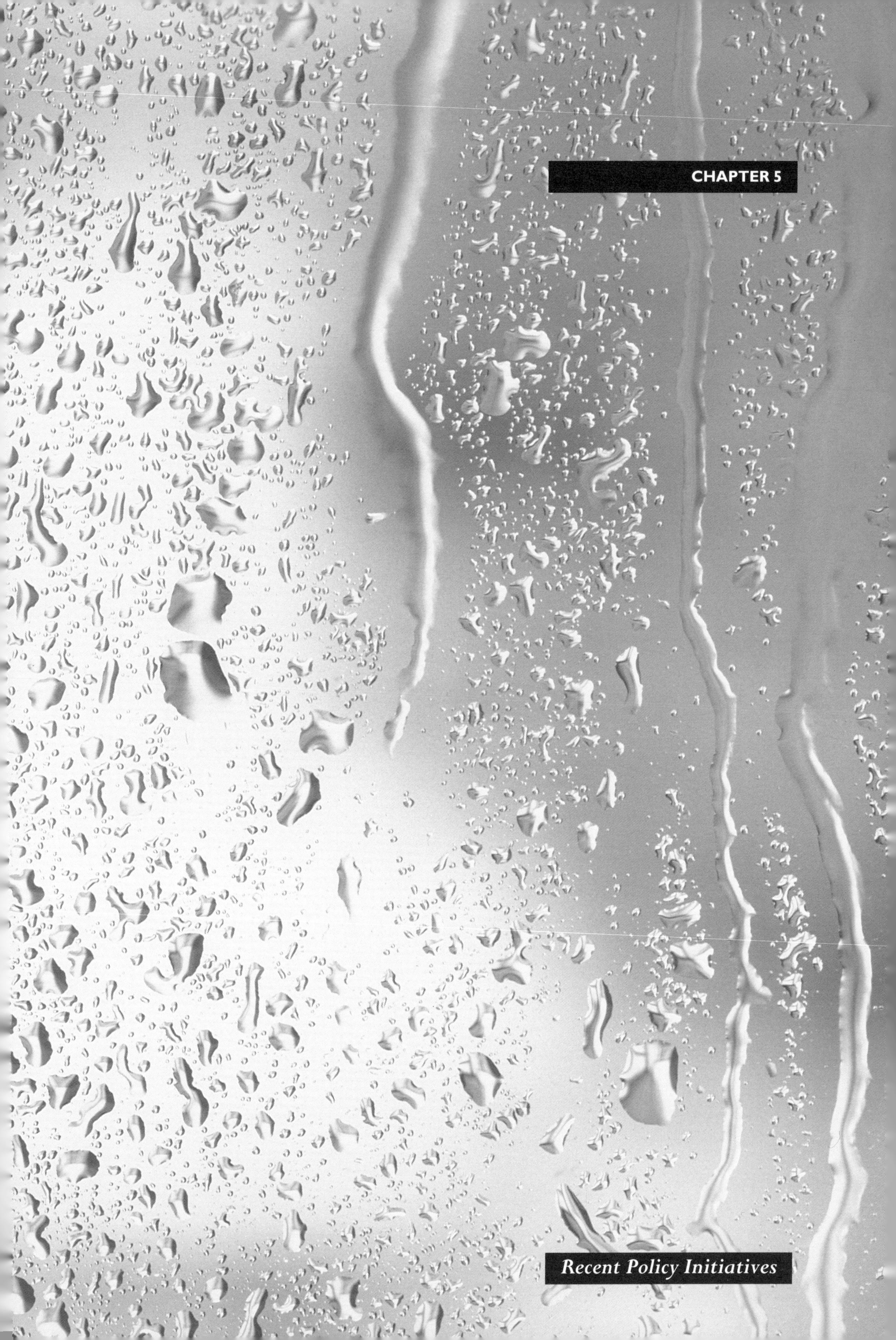

# CHAPTER 5

# *Recent Policy Initiatives*

## THE PATIENTS' CHARTER

56 In reaffirming the rights of all individuals to receive high quality health care, the principles outlined in The Patients' Charter clearly have implications for purchasers and providers of services for homeless mentally ill people. For example, the right to be registered with a GP, a major point of entry into the mental health services, often proves to be an insurmountable barrier to health care for homeless people. The fundamental right to be treated with equal dignity and respect and the right to be discharged appropriately are also frequently denied to homeless mentally ill people.

## THE NHS AND COMMUNITY CARE ACT 1990

57 The NHS and Community Care Act 1990 outlines the major reforms that shape the way health and social services are now planned and provided. The community care part of this legislation identifies social services departments as the lead agency responsible for assessing the needs of, and providing support to, people who are vulnerable because of ill health or age, who need care and support to live independently.

58 One of the major contemporary concerns, raised with the HAS by a variety of organisations and practitioners, about the effect of current community care policies on homeless people, is that the Act does not recognise that some in need of care have no place to live. Also, the Act presumes that those who need services can be or are easily in touch with them. Concerns were expressed about the different ways in which agencies interpret residency and whether this prevents homeless people from gaining access to assessment and care.

59 On the positive side, the policy of care in the community has focused attention on the joint planning of services involving local authorities, health authorities and the voluntary sector. It has succeeded in bringing interest to bear on the needs of homeless people. Consequently, the authorities in a number of areas have set up joint planning teams for homeless people or have identified the need for existing teams (eg mental health teams) to deal with homeless people. A task for the future is that of monitoring the influence of joint planning on services to disadvantaged service users.

60 While the health service reforms make no specific reference to the needs of homeless people, they do offer a range of opportunities for giving priority to the needs of disadvantaged groups.

61 The separation of purchasers and providers and the introduction of contracts has required a cultural change in the NHS. Funding is now given to purchasers to buy the services that most effectively meet the needs of their local population. As purchasers should be giving priority to those in greatest need within their local population, it is to be hoped that homeless mentally ill people will benefit in the longer term.

62 *Purchasing For Health* (Department of Health, 1993) identified three goals for purchasers (Table 1).

*Table 1*

| Goals for Purchasers |
|---|
| They must buy to: |
| • Improve people's health by targeting resources on effective ways of delivering clinical care and promoting health |
| • Improve the quality of health care, making it more responsive to the wishes and needs of people |
| • Ensure that as many people as possible receive high quality care from what available resources can provide |

63  The document aims to facilitate better working between purchasers and providers, and to improve the involvement of users and clinicians in service development. It identifies seven stepping stones to good purchasing, seven imperatives for effective contracting and guiding principles for measuring success. These approaches and how they apply to homeless mentally ill people are described in detail in Part C of this report.

## THE HEALTH OF THE NATION

64  Launched in England in 1992, this strategic initiative identified mental illness as one of the five key areas for health improvement. The White Paper proposed quantified targets for reducing suicides and unexplained deaths and an unquantified target for improving the health and social functioning of people with mental health problems (Table 2).

*Table 2*

| Health of the Nation Targets for Mental Illness |
|---|
| • To improve significantly the health and social functioning of mentally ill people |
| • To reduce the overall suicide rate* by at least 15% by the year 2000 (from 11.1 per 100,000 population in 1990 to no more than 9.4) |
| • To reduce the suicide rate* of severely mentally ill people by at least 33% by the year 2000 (from the estimate of 15% in 1990 to no more than 10%) |
| *Includes unexplained deaths |

65  Given the high prevalence of mental health problems and the enhanced risk of suicide and deliberate self-harm in people who are homeless (see chapter 6), the probability of achieving these goals will be greatly improved if multi-agency strategies take into account the specific needs of homeless people. This report informs the initiation and monitoring of these strategies.

## SUPERVISED DISCHARGES AND SUPERVISION REGISTERS

66  In 1994, in response to recent tragedies, the Secretary of State for Health announced a ten-point plan for improving care in the community in England. Much of that plan built upon previous policy (for example, the Health of the Nation). However, a key policy initiative, with important consequences for the care of seriously mentally ill people who are also homeless, was the establishment of local supervision registers and a prospective power of supervised discharge. Implementation of the latter requires primary legislation and, as this report is written, a Bill is before the Houses of Parliament.

67    Supervision registers are intended to include existing users of mental health services at risk of serious self-harm or neglect or of causing serious harm to others. In England, best practice would indicate incorporating the introduction of such registers with the implementation of the Care Programme Approach and improving practice with respect to Section 117 of the Mental Health Act 1983. The introduction of supervision registers may have important consequences for those homeless people, coming under the care of specialist mental health services, who fall into one of the 'at risk' categories. Registers (and the associated policy) should ensure the allocation of a keyworker and a co-ordinated care plan for such vulnerable mentally ill people, which will improve the continuity of their care.

## WALES

68    *Mental Illness - A Strategy for Wales* (Welsh Office, 1989) provides a broad framework for the development of comprehensive mental health care throughout the Principality. *The Protocol for Investment in Health Gain - Mental Health* (Welsh Health Planning Forum, 1993) offers detailed guidance to NHS commissioners and local authorities. It builds upon the earlier strategy and, in doing so, makes specific references to homeless mentally ill people. Homelessness is identified as a significant socio-economic factor linked to mental ill-health; the provision of appropriate housing is seen as an area of potential health gain for homeless people. The section in the protocol which deals with the development of a people-centred service stresses the importance of access, flexibility, responsiveness and choice. Such a people-centred service must be targeted at everyone who needs it, including people who are homeless. The protocol offers a valuable model to all managers responsible for formulating strategies for mental health.

## PROPOSED CHANGES IN HOUSING LEGISLATION

69    In January 1994, the Government published a Green Paper entitled *Access to Local Authority and Housing Association Tenancies*. At the time of publication of this review, the Government has announced that a Housing Bill is to be one of the core Bills it plans to include in the 1995-96 Parliamentary session. It is expected that the main proposals in the Green Paper are likely to be included in the new Housing Bill. These proposals would result in the alteration of parts of the current legislation relating to homeless people.

70    Originally, the proposals were that local authorities would only have a duty towards people who were literally roofless and that the duty would only be to secure them temporary accommodation, probably in the private sector. The waiting list would become the only route to a permanent local authority or housing association tenancy. There was no proposal to change the priority groups as defined by the current legislation in the Green Paper. The duty on local authorities will be to secure accommodation for a minimum of one year.

71    Subsequently, the proposal that only people who are roofless should be entitled to help has been modified. It seems likely that people in refuges and direct access and hostel accommodation will also qualify for help. It appears that Government plans to tighten the rules relating to people who are considered to have intentionally made themselves homeless (intentionality) and to urge authorities to investigate thoroughly the

circumstances in which someone has become homeless from the home of friends or relatives.

72     The HAS is aware that concerns have been expressed by some agencies about these proposals, with reference to homeless people with mental health problems, because they are seen to reduce the limited safety net that is available through the Housing Act 1985. The Government has said it will ensure that housing is made available to some *vulnerable people who cannot be expected to make their own arrangements.* However, experience has shown that homeless people with mental health problems are already excluded by the interpretation of vulnerability used by some local authorities. Any narrowing of the set of people that is covered by the term *vulnerable* could lead to an increase in street homelessness. If the duty of the local authorities is simply to secure homeless people accommodation, rather than allowing the opportunity for people to settle into their own permanent independent accommodation, this route into housing is likely to be even less appropriate for people experiencing mental health problems. Agencies working with homeless people have expressed fears that vulnerable people, who currently live with relatives where relationships may be breaking down, may not be treated as having an urgent need for re-housing even though mental illness may be closely linked to such breakdown.

## THE HOUSING IMPLICATIONS OF THE CRIMINAL JUSTICE AND PUBLIC ORDER ACT 1994

73     The Criminal Justice and Public Order Act 1994 became law in November 1994. There are two aspects of that Act which have implications for the groups of people with which this review is concerned.

74     The Act makes it a criminal offence not to vacate property after a landlord has gained a court order. It is predicted that this could lead to evictions and result in the homelessness of substantial numbers of people.

75     This Act also removes the duty on local authorities to provide sites for travellers. Fewer sites might result in there being more unlawful encampments, with the consequent lack of access to services and attendant health problems. The penalties for illegal camping will be much more severe, potentially causing serious problems for travellers. Evicted and homeless travellers will need to be placed in temporary accommodation while their status is investigated before being rehoused by local authorities.

# CHAPTER 6

A Survey of the
Literature - Findings
in England and Wales
and the USA

## INTRODUCTION

76   Before discussing potential service responses to meeting the mental health care needs of homeless people, it is important to identify who is covered by the term *homeless people* and to highlight what is already known about the characteristics of this group of people. Gathering this information is not an easy task and it is difficult to give totally reliable figures. However, where possible, references are given to allow readers opportunities to explore the sources of the data in more detail.

## SOME BASIC FACTS AND FIGURES

77   Combining data from pressure groups and official statistics, it is estimated that between one and two million people are homeless in Great Britain. While the actual number is debatable, all sources agree that homelessness is rising at a significant rate and that is has doubled between 1980 and 1990 (Scott, 1992). At different times, it was calculated that about 50,000 people were sleeping rough in England (Matthews, 1982) and that at least 100,000 homeless people in all settings were of less than 25 years of age (McKechnie, 1988). Furthermore, as described later, the mean age of the homeless population is falling and the gender distribution is changing with the rate of increase in the number of homeless women (with and without children) outstripping that of men.

78   Government statistics for 1992 record that local authorities accepted 148,250 households as homeless, a threefold increase since 1978. These figures represent one third of the number of people who applied as homeless for accommodation in that year under the provisions of the Housing Act 1985.

79   Overall, inner London still has the highest incidence of registered homeless people with 4.0 per 1,000 households against 1.6 per 1,000 for the rest of England. In England, of the 12 local authorities ranked highest for homeless registrations, six were in London. Although London has always been seen as the most problematic area in terms of homelessness, about two-thirds of homeless people live outside the capital. Furthermore, the rate of increase during the last decade was actually 50% greater outside London, both in metropolitan and non-metropolitan districts. The greatest proportional increases were in the Midlands, Humberside and Yorkshire.

80   Homelessness has frequently been perceived as purely an urban problem. While it is true that the absolute number of homeless people in rural areas is small, the problem has worsened considerably with about 12% of the total national homeless population being located in country areas. Single people in rural areas are also less likely to be made priority acceptances for housing (10% of such cases) than single people living in urban areas (17% of priority acceptances).

## DEFINITIONS OF HOMELESSNESS

81   Attempts to calculate the numbers of homeless people throw into sharp relief the complex problem of what constitutes homelessness. Stern et al (1989), in comparing and contrasting some 40 definitions of homelessness, surmised that the high level of disagreement partly derives from confusion about whether *homelessness* refers simply to a lack of adequate shelter or to the lack of a *home*. The latter concept incorporates more subtle social

relationships as well as the physical structure of the accommodation as the quote at the head of chapter one illustrates.

82    At present, the currently enforced legal definition of homelessness, as stated in the Housing Act 1985, includes the groups of people with which this review is concerned (Table 3).

*Table 3*

| Housing Act 1985 Definitions of Homelessness |
| --- |
| People are considered to be homeless if they and those members of their family with whom they normally live: |
| • have no accommodation that they are entitled to occupy; |
| • have a home but are unable to gain entry to it; |
| • have a home but are in danger of violence from someone living there; |
| • have accommodation which is moveable (for example, a caravan or houseboat) and they have nowhere to place it. |

83    People are considered to be threatened with homelessness if they are likely to fall into one of the above categories within 28 days.

## CLASSIFYING HOMELESS POPULATIONS

84    From this definition of homelessness, it becomes apparent that there are many sub-groups within this population: the *street person* stereotypes of the male *skid-row alcoholic*, the female *bag lady*, or more recently, young people in *cardboard city*. The most visible group actually represents a small minority (probably only 1 in 100) of all homeless people (Scott, 1992). Homeless people have never been a homogeneous group (Drake et al, 1982), but the increase in the size of the population has been accompanied by further changes in their characteristics (Lowry, 1987). The problem is best regarded as a *home to homelessness continuum* (Austerberry and Watson, 1986) within which different subgroups or levels of homelessness can be identified. Several attempts have been made to achieve a systematic sub-classification of the homeless population.

85    One suggested comprehensive attempt to define broad categories of homelessness, along a continuum from those at risk of becoming homeless to those living rough, is found in the Greve Report published in 1986 (Greve, J. et al, *Homelessness in London*, GLC Research Team). The recommendations of that report as to the categories of people who are considered as homeless are listed below:

   •    People literally without a roof over their heads, including those sleeping rough.

   •    People in accommodation specifically provided on a temporary basis for homeless people (hotels, bed and breakfast lodgings).

   •    People with insecure or impermanent tenure. (This includes: other [self-referred] hotel or bed and breakfast residents; licensees and those in holiday lettings; those in tied accommodation who lose or change jobs; private tenants under notice to quit; squatters; and licensed occupants of short-life housing.)

- People subject to discrimination in respect of housing.

- People shortly to be released or discharged from institutional accommodation including hospitals, prisons, community or foster homes or other hostels who have no existing alternative accommodation or household to rejoin.

- Households in which people are sharing involuntarily (which appeared to be the case for the majority of homeless people in the 1981 Census).

- Individuals or groups living within existing households where either:

  - relationships with the rest of the household;

  - living conditions;

  are highly unsatisfactory and intolerable for any extended period.

- Individuals or groups living within existing households whose relationships and conditions are tolerable but where there is a clear preference to live separately.

- Individuals who have accommodation, but where the occupancy would lead to a risk of domestic violence towards them or other dependents.

86  These groupings present clear implications for people with mental health problems. In many cases, their family relationships may be fragile or at breaking point and some form of independent supported housing may offer better prospects of improved mental health. In other cases, homeless people will develop a pattern of repeated moves from one insecure address to another, resulting in their losing contact with mental health services and the community in general. These are highly vulnerable people who manage, all too frequently, to remain hidden to service providers, in both urban and rural areas.

87  A system, based on geographical location, was suggested by Austerberry and Watson (1986) and also by Roth and Bean (1986). Creating divisions within a continuum is always arbitrary. However, this approach has some benefit for researchers working with homeless populations as it allows groups within a location to be targeted (without making assumptions about the characteristics and needs of the groups). This system recognises the fact that service developments have often been targeted at individuals residing in a specific setting. The four geographical categories identified by Austerberry and Watson (1986) are:

- Street people or those sleeping rough.

- Residents of shelters and hostels for homeless people.

- Residents of hotels or bed and breakfast accommodation - often families in temporary accommodation.

- Other unique situations, eg people without accommodation who are staying with family or friends, squatters, travellers.

88 The proportion of homeless people in each of these sub-groups in a locality can be calculated approximately and their characteristics can be assessed. However, it must be acknowledged that a major disadvantage of this classification is that it offers a static portrait of a situation which, in reality, is one of a state of flux as people frequently move from one form of homeless accommodation to another.

*"People are in cars, buses, caravans and tents."*

*Quote from user*

89 The teams undertaking the service visits for this review, worked within a broad definition of homelessness and observed a number of distinct groups which extended the list above.

- Street homeless people

- Travellers - New Age and traditional

- Single parents, including residents of refuges

- Refugees

- Homeless people from black and ethnic communities

- Homeless people in rural areas

- People in insecure accommodation, eg bed-sits, squats, friends' floors

- Psychiatric inpatients who had no home to go to

- Homeless elderly people

90 This is not a finite list and there is likely to be some overlap between the categories. As noted in this and previous studies (Department of Health, 1994; Royal College of Physicians, 1994), the significant need, shared by all homeless people, is for access to appropriate, affordable housing.

91 Given the inherent limitations of classifying homelessness, it is instructive to identify the roots of, and pathways to, homelessness.

## PATHWAYS TO HOMELESSNESS

92 The pathways to homelessness are often complex but there are a number of frequently quoted routes, which involve the following factors and processes.

### Economic Factors

While unemployment contributes to the size of the homelessness problem, it should be noted that a significant minority of homeless people are employed, indicating that a key issue is the shortage of affordable housing. In this country, the number of new council or housing association homes built in 1986 fell to only 25% of the 1975 level. There was also a 60% reduction in the amount of accommodation available for rent (Mariasy, 1987). By virtue of their impaired earning power, people with moderate or severe mental illness are less likely to become homeowners and thus they tend to be restricted to rented accommodation. Between 1987 and 1993, 316,560 homes were repossessed. In 1993, a further 200,000 homeowners were more than six months in arrears with mortgage repayments and in danger of losing their homes through repossession.

### Social Factors

Forty-two per cent of homeless people put their situation down to the fact that parents, relatives or friends cannot, or will not, accommodate them. Marital disharmony was identified as the cause in about 20% of cases (Central Statistics Office, 1989).

### Deinstitutionalisation

In America, deinstitutionalisation of psychiatric patients accounted for 20-30% of the homeless population (Rivlin, 1986). However, the situation in the UK is very different and studies have shown that only 1-2% of long-stay patients who have subsequently left psychiatric hospitals have become homeless.

Preclusive admission policies mean that many young undomiciled adults with chronic mental illness have had only sporadic contact with mental health services and have never been institutionalised.

Deinstitutionalisation in its wider sense obviously plays a significant role in the problem. Many people become homeless after leaving a diverse range of institutional settings.

### Intentional Homelessness

Very few people choose to become homeless. Local authorities are required to assess whether someone has made themselves intentionally homeless, although, in practice, this involves deciding whether people have left accommodation unnecessarily rather than having made a choice to become homeless. Studies of people in hostels show that fewer than 4% of respondents chose to have no home.

93    Although these themes represent the most frequently identified primary reasons for becoming homeless, it must be emphasised that homelessness is rarely the result of a single event. Merves (1986) describes three processes by which people become homeless:

### Skid or Slide

This is the culmination of several events leading to a downward spiral (eg the circumstances of a person who left home following the death of a parent and moved into rented accommodation, then failed to cope with bereavement and did not go to work, consequently losing his or her job, resulting in inability to pay the rent, loss of accommodation before staying with friends until they felt they could no longer offer a room).

### Periodic or Cyclical

This is represented by a constant juggling of limited resources leading to intermittent periods of homelessness as a survival strategy (eg an individual with a drug-related problem who moves from parents to a treatment unit, then to temporary accommodation and then back to parents).

### Critical Juncture

This describes a major change point when people directly choose to leave a situation (eg one of domestic violence) in an attempt to take control of their lives.

## CHARACTERISTICS OF HOMELESS POPULATIONS

94    This section reviews demographic trends, examines the mental health problems of homeless people and concludes by highlighting other factors associated with the state of being homeless.

## Demographic Trends

95 Studies published prior to the 1980s identified the homeless population as comprising predominantly single middle-aged males (Freeman et al, 1979; Priest, 1976). Surveys undertaken in the last decade, which have sampled homeless populations from a wider variety of settings, suggest a rather different demographic composition. Importantly, these studies show that age and gender vary significantly across the different settings (Department of Health, 1994). For example, male hostel residents in Britain are predominantly aged under 45 years and their mean age has fallen since the mid-1960s (O'Neill, 1989; Stark et al, 1989). Female hostel residents have not been studied as extensively, but surveys reveal wide differences. Marshall and Reed (1992) found that the mean age of women using one London direct access hostel was 52 years. However, Scott (1991-94) interviewed women using government-run resettlement units and temporary accommodation and found their mean age to be 33 years. These differences, while highlighting the problem of trying to generalise from small studies to the wider population, also have implications for planning interventions. Marshall and Reed's study found a very high prevalence of psychotic illness in the women interviewed, while Scott (1991) showed different patterns of mental health problems among younger and older women, with less psychotic illness but higher levels of drug and alcohol problems in young people.

96 More extensive surveys have been undertaken in London. The organisation Access to Health (1992) undertook a systematic survey of individuals in five settings of homelessness. It found that, while 45% of all the homeless people identified were aged 15-44 years, the age distribution varied considerably, with 40% of those in temporary accommodation being of less than 15 years of age, nearly 60% of individuals in hostels being 15-44 years old and about 40% of those sleeping out were over 45 years of age. A separate study by Victor (1992) of homeless people in temporary accommodation in the former North West Thames Region demonstrated that 72% of those interviewed were aged 16-34 years old.

97 A census in Sheffield showed that up to 25% of the single homeless population was female (George et al, 1991). While about one in seven of street people are women, and 60-80% of hostel bed spaces are allocated to men, females comprise 60-70% of homeless people housed in temporary accommodation (Victor, 1992). Many of the women (up to 70% in some studies) in the latter setting are accompanied by children. In two small studies in Newcastle, it was found that up to 28% of those using temporary accommodation were two parent families, and 36% were one parent families (Scott & Boustead, 1990; Scott, 1994).

## Ethnicity

98 There are considerable difficulties in trying to draw a national picture of the ethnic composition of the homeless population. Much depends upon which groups within that population, and which parts of the country, are being examined and it is impossible to make general statements on this aspect of homelessness. Nonetheless, there are some findings from a number of research studies conducted in London which have relevance to other urban areas, including inner city and sea port locations.

99   The Living in Temporary Accommodation survey in 1989 was a national survey of homeless people placed by local authorities and people who placed themselves in temporary accommodation. This found that homelessness among black and minority ethnic groups was a particular problem in London. Of those people interviewed in London, 43% came from African, African-Caribbean and Asian ethnic groups. This is a far higher proportion than their representation in the wider population. Surveys in Hackney and Newham, and the recent evaluation of the Rough Sleepers Initiative all indicate that over one-third of homeless people were categorised as African, African-Caribbean or Black Other. Within those groups in the Rough Sleepers Initiative survey, over half were women, compared to one-fifth in the white population. Homeless black people were younger - only 5% were over the age of 35, compared to the population of white homeless people in which over 50% is aged over 35. Hidden homelessness is a more common feature for black people, in that 30% had experience of sleeping rough compared with the 80% of the white population who had done so.

100  These figures should be compared with the recent study of health status in the residents of resettlement units for men in which the vast majority (92%) were white.

101  Where monitoring has included Irish people as an ethnic minority, they are very significantly over-represented in the homeless population. In London Boroughs, the percentage of the population which is Irish varies between 2% and 7%. Surveys have shown that up to 30% of street homeless people are Irish and that the largest group using severe weather shelters in December-January 1990-91 was of Irish origin. CARA 1991, London. *Access to Housing for Irish Single Homeless People.*

**Status and Skills**

102  The majority of homeless people are single or separated (Burt & Cohen, 1989). Hostel surveys show that less than one-third of the males had ever married (Stark et al, 1989) and this is approximately half the rate for domiciled men. Female hostel residents are more likely to have married than their male counterparts (Scott, 1991).

103  As Stearn (1987) points out, homeless does not mean rootless. Fifty to sixty per cent of homeless people remain in a single city for more than one year, and among resettlement services for users, over 50% of men and women had stayed within a relatively local area (radius 20-30 miles) for more than five of the previous 10 years.

104  In Britain, few homeless people have any paid employment (Herzberg, 1987; Royal College of Physicians, 1994; Stark et al, 1989). Reviews of previous histories have shown that most homeless men have been employed at some time, but that their work records were unstable; for example, 30% had failed to retain a job for more than two years (Stark et al, 1989). There are significant differences in skills levels between homeless and domiciled people, with the majority of the former having only ever held unskilled or labouring jobs (Fernandez, 1984; Stark et al, 1989). The reduced demand for low-skilled labourers makes these individuals particularly vulnerable to unemployment.

*"It became clear, from their view, that for a vulnerable black person, the homeless circuit would be dangerous - racism, aggression and violence could be experienced to a greater degree than for a white person. . . "*

Quote from user visitor report

105 It was previously noted that homeless people tend to have had a minimum schooling (Fischer et al, 1986; Herzberg, 1987) and, in one study, 11-17% of the men interviewed had attended special schools (Stark et al, 1989). Interestingly, Scott (1991) recently found contrasting results with 37% of women hostel dwellers in London reporting that they had stayed in school until at least 18 years. A similar figure was reported by Bassuk et al (1986) in the USA. However, only in a very few cases had educational attainment translated into occupational skills. The majority of the women reported records of unstable employment in semi-skilled or unskilled jobs.

## Mental Illness and Homelessness

106 Much has been written on homelessness and mental illness. However, estimates of the nature, extent and severity of these disorders vary considerably. The lack of consistency in the results obtained reflects problems in undertaking this research. The most recent studies suggest that as many as 50% of the total homeless population may have some form of mental disorder (Scott, 1992). In Britain (Victor, 1992), it is estimated that at least twice as many homeless as domiciled people have some form of mental health problem and that, in general, their disorders are of a more severe nature. Disorders may be both a cause and a consequence of homelessness and it has been noted that mental illness tends to worsen as homelessness continues.

107 The two groups of homeless people that have been investigated most frequently are those residents of hostels and shelters who were willing to take part in prevalence studies or those of no fixed abode who were attending hospital facilities. Other research on homeless individuals in other temporary accommodation, in food lines, on the streets, or presenting to travellers aid groups, suggests levels of psychiatric morbidity as high as, or in excess of, the findings of the studies of the first two groups. It is not surprising to note that street people were particularly likely to show high levels of delusion, disorientation, withdrawal and avoidance of contact with services (Fischer & Breakey, 1986).

108 Recently, Scott (1992) undertook a review of research on homelessness and mental illness. Studies of hostel and shelter populations have suggested that the overall prevalence of psychosis was 30-50%, with the majority of individuals in this group suffering from schizophrenia. Most of the subjects interviewed had a history of previous hospitalisation and many demonstrated high levels of associated psycho-social problems which significantly impeded their day-to-day functioning (Marshall and Reed, 1992; Stark et al, 1989). Evidence suggests that homeless mentally ill women have had much less experience of institutional living (either hospitals or prison) than the men (Burt & Cohen, 1989). Scott (1991) also found that female hostel residents with mental health problems generally functioned at a higher level than their male counterparts. However, there may also be an age-related effect as Marshall and Reed (1992) found higher levels of psychiatric morbidity in their sample of older female hostel residents, compared to Scott's studies (1991-1994) in which the women were, on average, about 20 years younger.

109 Alcohol and/or drug misuse were also significant problems among hostel residents, occurring in 9-63%. It is estimated that the rate of alcohol misuse in homeless people is three to five times higher than that of the general population. In Britain, it has been demonstrated that co-morbidity of

alcohol-related problems and major psychiatric disorders occurs in at least one-fifth of hostel residents (Stark et al, 1989). Overall, drug misuse is becoming a more frequent feature in younger hostel users (Stark et al, 1989; Scott, 1991). The prevalence of alcohol misuse is lower in females (Scott, 1994) but drug misuse may be equally prevalent in young females as in young males (Scott, 1994).

110   Thirty to eighty per cent of homeless individuals interviewed reported current psychological distress as measured on the General Health Questionnaire (GHQ, Goldberg 1972). In Scott's (1991) study of female resettlement unit users, younger women reported current distress more often than drug, alcohol or other major mental health problems. In one study (Linn et al, 1989), distress in the homeless population was particularly correlated with unemployment, greater alcohol intake, poor physical health, lack of social support and anxieties related to difficulties in gaining access to medical services. The rate of deliberate self-harm among homeless people may be seven times that of the general population.

*"He said he was having several problems - isolation, loneliness, the inability to make relationships, suicidal thoughts, depression and severe breakdown - he felt life was hardly worth living."*

Quote from user visitor report

111   Personality problems were not investigated in all studies. Stark et al (1989) commented on the difficulty of assessing personality in their sample and omitted such data because of poor reliability. Where personality was assessed, the prevalence of disorder varied considerably. In Scott's surveys (1991-1994), about one-third of the men and women demonstrated evidence of personality dysfunction, but in only a few was the disorder regarded as severe.

112   Studies of organic impairment have found rates of less than one in 10 except among the long-stay population of resettlement units. Stark et al (1989) found evidence of significant cognitive impairment in over one-third of the men interviewed, and 75% of those with impairment were under the age of 65 years. About half of those with organic impairment had a history of drug or alcohol-related problems.

113   Maitra (1982) reviewed the reasons for the attendance at an accident and emergency department by 73 homeless people. One-third presented with alcohol-related problems and one-fifth presented with an 'acute crisis', often following an episode of deliberate self-harm. Information gathered retrospectively suggested that 13-16% of casualty attendances by homeless males related to alcohol or drug withdrawal problems (Kelly, 1985; Stark et al, 1989). Access to GP and other primary healthcare services is a widespread problem particularly with regard to full registration.

114   The problems of homeless families and their children requires research. Scott and Boustead (1991) found that the parents accompanied by children scored higher on the General Health Questionnaire than other people living in temporary accommodation. In a study in London of homeless adults in hotel accommodation (65% of whom were accompanied by dependent children), Victor (1992) found the prevalence of mental morbidity to be more than twice that of the domiciled population of that region.

115   Children living with their parents in hostels for homeless people are also at risk. Nearly half of the under-fives showed at least one developmental delay. At school, one-third were attending special classes. The Health

Visitors Association and the Bayswater Project confirm that children suffer physically, emotionally and educationally when living in bed and breakfast accommodation. This research showed a high incidence of depression, disturbed sleep, poor eating, overactivity, bed-wetting and soiling, toilet training problems, temper tantrums and aggression (Drennan & Stearn, 1986; Health Visitors Association, 1989). Single mothers may be victims of domestic violence, and children may have experienced violence or sexual abuse. These families may move addresses frequently, or be forced out of lodgings all day. Their findings have service implications here, and indicate the need for tracking systems.

## Other Associated Difficulties

116 Homeless people often report a number of other significant health and social difficulties. Some of the most frequent issues are briefly reviewed here. It is noteworthy that homeless mentally ill people appear to have a greater prevalence of all these problems.

### Physical Health Problems

117 The homeless lifestyle contributes to increased morbidity rates and mortality rates are increased at least threefold in homeless as opposed to domiciled populations (Royal College of Physicians, 1994). Seven to thirteen per cent of individuals interviewed see prior ill-health as the cause of their homelessness. Despite this, only 20-50% of hostel residents seek or receive treatment for any of their reported problems.

118 At least 25% of shelter occupants have one or more significant physical health problems. Co-morbidity for physical illness and alcohol problems or physical and mental illness occurs in about one-third of the hostel residents. In men and women, the length of time of homelessness is associated with increased prevalence of physical illness. Chronic ill-health affects up to 15% of homeless people under 30 years of age and over 50% of those aged 50 years or more (Stark et al, 1989).

119 Homeless people often show particular patterns of morbidity that require greater than average care (Royal College of Physicians, 1994; Shanks, 1983). Lack of access to primary care often leads to high usage of accident and emergency facilities (Maitra, 1982; Victor et al, 1989; Williams & Allen, 1989). Those attending casualty departments report a disproportionate prevalence (14-33%) of traumatic injuries. Fifty per cent are cases of repeated trauma, and in many this is the result of physical or sexual assault (Kelly, 1985). High prevalence rates are also recorded for infections, particularly of the respiratory tract (with 5-15% of individuals studied having active tuberculosis), scabies and lice, cellulitis, peripheral vascular disease, leg ulcers and frostbite.

120 Research on other homeless groups is less readily available, but one London hospital reported that one-tenth of its beds was used by families living in bed and breakfast accommodation (Victor et al, 1989). Women in such settings are at greater risk of problems during pregnancy and are more likely to require hospitalisation than their domiciled counterparts. Children are at particular risk of infection (especially that resulting in diarrhoea) while burns and scalds seem to be a specific hazard (Victor et al, 1989).

### Early Adversity and Lack of Social Networks

121  Childhood histories reveal that placements away from the family home in institutional settings are a frequent feature of homeless populations. Stark et al (1989) found that 37% of male long-stay residents in resettlement units came from broken homes and a further 15% had been separated from their parents for an extended period of time. O'Neill (1988) found that, in younger resettlement unit users, 44% of those under 20 years and 32% of those aged 20-29 years had spent at least six months in local authority care. Many went to the hostels immediately after discharge from local authority care. Recent studies of women who were residents of shelters revealed that one-third may have been sexually or physically abused during childhood and two-thirds reported major family disruptions.

*"Many people who are homeless and have mental health problems are the product of the child care system."*

*Quote from user visitor report*

122  Homeless men and women are marginalised from society. This disaffiliation may be both a cause and a consequence of their homelessness. One-third to a half of all homeless people staying in hostels or resettlement units had no recognisable social contacts with family or friends, although women appeared to retain their networks more successfully than men (Scott, 1991). Among homeless mentally ill people, however, social networks are restricted with 60-90% having no contacts. Where contacts do exist, they are often superficial and restricted to people in close proximity, ie other hostel residents (Stark et al, 1989). The latter study also suggested that the longer people are homeless the fewer social contacts they retain.

123  Refugees are part of the homeless population in many urban areas. Numbers are difficult to ascertain because people may be hidden through, for instance, living with friends in overcrowded dwellings. There may be particular health needs specific to this group. A proportion will be suffering from post-traumatic stress disorders as the result of war and torture. They will have different religious and cultural needs and may speak little or no English.

124  People from black and other ethnic communities are increasingly becoming homeless. Even when living in reasonable housing however, they are known to under-use mental health services either from a deep sense of alienation and perception of racism among providers, or from ignorance of access to services, often compounded by language barriers. Again, this has policy and practical implications for providers.

125  In rural areas, there are other aspects of homelessness. It is frequently a seasonal, migratory phenomenon, and rural homeless populations may include agricultural workers. The numbers may be so small in total that people may be virtually invisible but still have serious problems. Carers in rural communities may willingly, or otherwise, assume greater responsibility for looking after a mentally ill relative than their urban counterparts.

126  Conversely, many rural areas have large populations of travellers, both traditional and New Age. Many of these people would not necessarily describe themselves as homeless, but increasingly their life style and the impacts of the Criminal Justice and Public Order Act 1994 tend to render them vulnerable to homelessness and to problems of mental and physical ill-health.

127 Homeless elderly people present particular features. For example, they age more rapidly than the housed population, because of their poor health. They may have become homeless following a bereavement or loss of tied housing, and there will be a higher proportion of women in this age group. Again, there are specific service implications for commissioners and providers.

### Forensic Problems

*"The old cops are alright, the young ones have got something to prove"*

*"Police are head doers."*

*Quotes from users*

128 Early British studies found that 22-37% of homeless people had a criminal record (Berry & Orwin, 1966; Priest, 1976), while 18% had been in prison in the previous year (Tidmarsh & Wood, 1972). More recent surveys, by Stark et al (1989) and Weller et al (1987), show that about twice as many homeless people with past or present psychiatric problems had been imprisoned compared to those without a history of mental illness. Analysis of types of criminal activity suggests that offences against property or related to intoxication much exceed those for violence. Much of this offending occurs after people have become homeless. Serious offences are a cause for concern in a significant minority of males who are homeless (Weller et al, 1987).

# CHAPTER 7

Findings from the
Service Visits

## INTRODUCTION

129   The service visits, made by HAS teams, were to 10 very different locations in England and Wales. The findings enabled the steering committee for this project to build upon its familiarity with the issues of homelessness in general, and upon its earlier work of reviewing the existing research and recent experience of service provision.

130   The teams found that certain core concerns were raised in each of the places visited. These form the basis of this report. Nonetheless, a major aim of the service visits was to seek out examples of innovation and good practice. Specific instances of good practice are set out in chapter 16. Examples are provided of high quality strategic planning, service delivery, cross-agency liaison and innovative appointments. Some of these can be attributed to the availability of additional ring-fenced capital and revenue resources, but, importantly, a number of creative and effective measures were found which had been put into effect from existing resources. These offer useful models for other authorities to consider for their own localities.

131   The teams were all impressed by the high level of commitment shown by those staff in both the statutory and voluntary sectors who work with homeless mentally ill people. Their readiness to act as advocates for their patients and clients was commendable. The other side of this coin, however, was that often these workers were over-loaded and sometimes marginalised by their colleagues in other parts of the service.

## AWARENESS

132   The overall impression was that, with one or two obvious exceptions in the inner cities, homelessness was not an apparent major concern to service managers and professionals. This appeared to be attributable to a number of matters. In some areas, the number of people homeless was very low, and the issue of their health needs had not been raised. In other places, there was a serious lack of information about the size and nature of the homeless population, and little awareness of possible sources of information. In a few areas, the visiting teams formed the view that there was significant denial of homelessness coupled with a notion that it might be unwise to raise its profile for fear of presenting additional demands on services which already considered themselves under pressure. The need for a sound knowledge-base as the foundation for needs assessment and strategy is set out in chapter 10.

## THE VOLUNTARY SECTOR

133   The other major finding, common to all the areas visited, was the particular importance of the voluntary organisations in providing services for homeless people, including those with mental health problems. The significance of this lies in the traditional role of voluntary and charitable bodies in providing a range of services to people who are often not in contact with anyone else. Without idealising them too much, these agencies are able to offer accessible and acceptable services, and they were found to provide a range of facilities and types of care under one roof to meet the needs of homeless people for shelter, warmth, food, advice and health care in a seamless manner. Additionally, the voluntary sector is important because, as the visits showed, it frequently has a considerable amount of information on the whereabouts of homeless people, their

*"There is no evidence of homelessness because no-one wants to know . . ."*

Quote from user

patterns of need and the ways in which the local networks of services and facilities operate in practice.

134 The ways in which voluntary organisations relate to health and social services vary considerably. In some cases, there is a thriving and mature relationship based on mutual respect and knowledge of each other's roles and responsibilities. In such cases, there is participation in planning and collaboration in provision of services. Other cases, however, indicated that there appears to be little dialogue, coupled with elements of mistrust and ignorance. In some areas, very effective steps have been taken to promote the development of voluntary sector work with mentally ill people (less so with homeless people). In a few areas, nearly all the initiative for service development and delivery appears to be coming from the voluntary agencies which are seen to be driving strategy and leading provision. The best services are usually found in places in which the statutory and voluntary sectors are working in strong alliance.

135 Another factor identified in the visits is the marked absence, in strategic plans or the commissioning processes for services for this client group, of any mention of homelessness and mental illness. This reflects the general lack of hard information available to commissioners. Where particular research has been undertaken for the purposes of needs assessment, this is very valuable, especially when the findings are shared between the health and social services and housing department staff. The commissioning, purchasing and contracting processes also vary in their state of development, both generally and in relation to homeless mentally ill people as a particular client group. Given the importance of the voluntary sector as a major provider, this section highlights the implications for commissioners. In this report we stress the importance of commissioners investing their time in working with the non-statutory agencies to achieve realistic and relevant needs assessments, service specifications and contracts.

## SPECIALIST SERVICES

136 The service visits showed that the issue of whether mental health services for homeless people should be specially designated or provided as part of the mainstream of mental health care, both hospital and community-based, has not been addressed in many local services. The HAS visiting teams recognise the value of specialist services for this client group, but they also conclude that there is a danger of their becoming marginalised unless there is an accompanying intention to open up mainstream services to make them more accessible and welcoming to homeless people. The possibility of working through both short and longer-term strategies to achieve this aim is one which seems a helpful way forward. A particular advantage of specialist mental health services for homeless people, which was identified in the fieldwork, was the way in which specialist services appeared to have greater freedom to work in settings frequented by the client group, and to spend time developing a trusting relationship with people who are often isolated and suspicious.

## GENERAL PRACTITIONER SERVICES

137 The teams experienced problems in making contact with GPs during their visits. The overall response rate to the questionnaires sent out in advance to all GPs was low, and generally very few of them attended the meetings which were arranged. The questionnaire returns indicated a low level of

awareness of issues of homelessness or the housing status of their patients. In many cases, it appeared that primary healthcare workers did not know about the routes to specific services and agencies for homeless people.

138  Nonetheless, there were, in most areas, a few GPs who were committed to caring for homeless people, including those with alcohol-related or mental health problems. Often, these doctors worked on a sessional basis in day centres and drop-in facilities, or made special arrangements in their own surgeries. The role of family health services authorities varied in addressing the question of registration of homeless people. Some (mentioned in chapter 16) have taken a strong lead in encouraging GPs to overcome their reported reluctance to register homeless people. In East London, the practice of attracting GPs to work with homeless people through enhanced sessional fees, as well as through effective co-ordination by one of their colleagues, certainly bears further consideration.

## TRAVELLERS

139  Among the groups of people who may be included under the general category of being homeless, the HAS visiting teams found that travellers were perceived as presenting major issues for service provision in large parts of England and Wales. Their migratory way of life, with seasonal coming and going, for agricultural work or festivals, presented a challenge to many authorities. While many travellers would not have designated themselves as homeless, their needs for primary healthcare were very similar to those of other homeless people, though less was reported by clinicians about mental health problems in this group. Reference was made by local staff to increased demand upon drug misuse services by travellers, especially around festival periods, and to the difficulties this presented to service providers.

## THE CARE PROGRAMME APPROACH

140  Some of the service visits identified effective measures which authorities had initiated to ensure that homeless people with mental health problems were included in the care planning processes. The degree to which the Care Programme Approach was being implemented in England varies greatly and there are clearly particular difficulties in ensuring that homeless people benefit from planned packages of care as they leave hospital. Part of the problem appears to be the difficulty of integrating assessments made in pursuit of care in the community with the Care Programme Approach, and, since the need for some form of housing is paramount in these cases, much depends on the operational links with housing services. Where, as in the case of the London Borough of Barnet (see chapter 16) there is an inter-agency special needs housing panel for mentally ill people, the process works very well.

*"You have to go where they put you - away from friends and family . . ."*

*"Young people with an assured tenancy will still need support for 12 to 18 months."*

*"Once you get a bit better there's no day care."*

*Quotes from users*

## LINKS WITH HOUSING SERVICES

141  This is a major concern reported by nearly all the visiting teams. Where steps have been taken, as in Barnet, to develop mechanisms for collaboration, homeless people are likely to receive a co-ordinated response to their needs. Coterminous authority boundaries certainly help, but this feature is often not the case. Where social services and housing departments are integrated, there is a clear benefit to their homeless clients. During some visits, teams found that there was little or no

communication between the county social services department and district councils' housing departments. Current and future local government boundary changes and the establishment of unitary authorities in Wales and parts of England may well bring greater collaboration across services.

## SUMMARY

142  Overall, the major findings of the fieldwork are:

- Some excellent instances of good practice (chapter 16).

- A low level of professional and managerial awareness of homelessness.

- Lack of strategy in the commissioning and provision of services for homeless people.

- Problems in obtaining the necessary information on homelessness and homeless people.

- The strategic and operational importance of the voluntary sector.

- Problems of access to services.

- Problems for homeless people in registering with GPs and the provision of primary care.

- The challenges presented to commissioners and providers by mobile populations, ie travellers.

- Difficulties in implementing the Care Programme Approach.

- Under-developed collaboration with housing services.

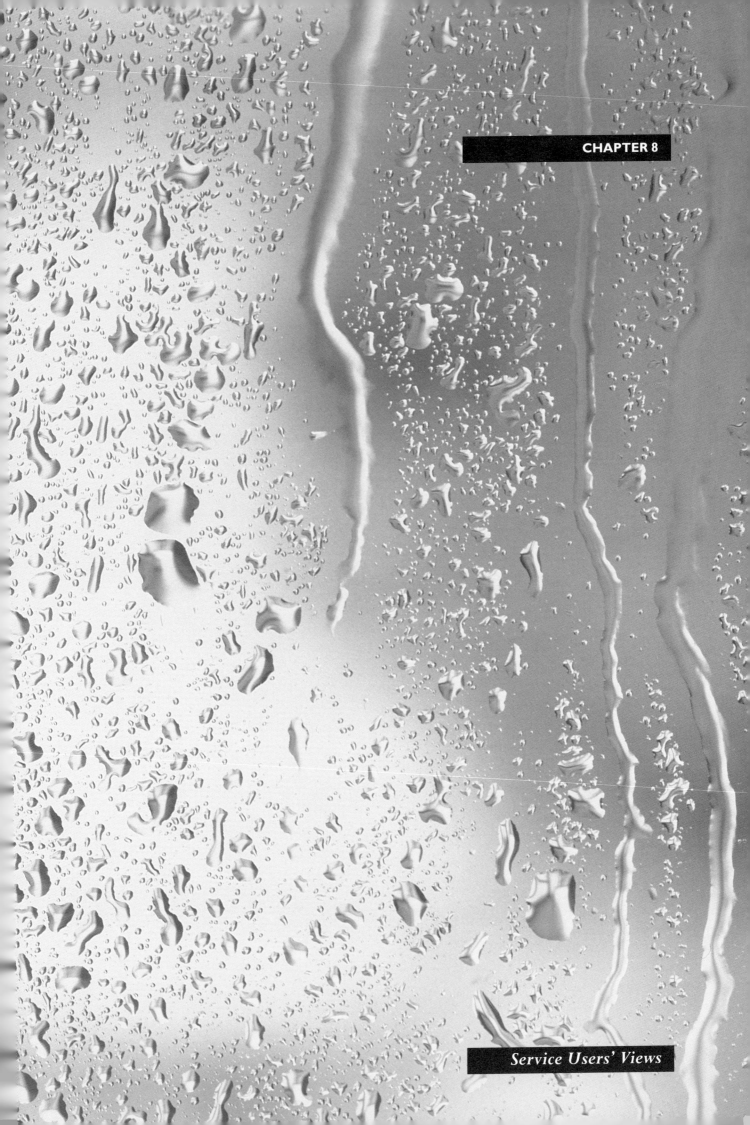

# CHAPTER 8

*Service Users' Views*

## LISTENING TO PATIENTS

143  In the Department of Health booklet, *Purchasing for Health - a Framework for Action*, the first guiding principle for measuring success is:

### Listen to Patients

*"...the whole idea of quality in the NHS is meaningless unless it focuses on issues that really matter to patients...."*

144  With this principle in mind, the HAS arranged for three groups of people who have had first-hand experience of using mental health services to visit the same areas as the HAS teams and talk directly with service users as well as voluntary organisations and professional staff. The three groups came from Wales, Bradford and Nottingham and the visits were scheduled so as to avoid service users visiting their own areas. The importance of this parallel programme of visits is that the users' findings highlight and reinforce favourable impressions about accessible and acceptable services and, at the same time, leave no room for complacency about the qualities of service which are inadequate and unacceptable to them.

*" We're really having our say, at last."*

*Quote from user*

145  This chapter is set out in a way which presents verbatim quotes from service users gained in the course of their interviews with other service users. It also includes, in the main text, summaries of the longer discussions with users, giving their personal perceptions of the issues that affect them. The aim of this chapter is to take the reader into the world of the homeless mentally ill people who were willing to share their experiences and opinions with people who had faced many of the same difficulties. These are their voices, and the authors of this report have attempted to present them with accuracy and an awareness of the need to balance the views of professional service providers with those on the receiving end. The chapter indicates some of the alienation and mistrust, the isolation and the anger which were expressed in the interviews. It also summarises the often expressed need for basic care, shelter, food and warmth as well as for health care.

## WHAT USERS SAY

146  Stigma is a major issue for people suffering from mental health problems. If, in addition, an individual also suffers the degradation of being homeless, the resulting erosion of self-esteem and sense of alienation from society is understandable, particularly since the majority of single homeless people with a mental health or substance misuse problem have experienced a relationship breakdown, or bereavement, or have previously used the residential child care system and have little or no family support.

147  Gaining access to services may be particularly difficult for homeless people as their voices are all too easily ignored. It appears from the HAS visits that few local authorities, health authorities or trusts have homelessness high on the agenda. Consequently, there are few specific services available to homeless people nationally, and the majority of those that do exist are based in the voluntary sector.

148  It appears that, despite the growing power of the user movement and the development of advocacy groups for people who are mentally ill, these

services tend to extend inadequately to homeless people who are mentally ill, and thus, their specific needs are rarely acknowledged or recognised.

149   A general lack of understanding by professional staff of the problems that have an impact on homeless people leads to their being confronted by attitudes which exacerbate their lack of self-worth and isolation and prevents them from seeking help.

*"People's ideas are pooh-poohed. They are afraid of being ostracised if they speak."*

*"How the hell they know what we want, I don't know; they never come and find out what we want."*

*"There's no concern for human misery and suffering, only monetary concerns."*

*"We need love, friendship and something more than a depressing hole like this..."*

*Quotes from users of the service*

### Resources for Homeless People

150   The visiting teams found that, despite there being large numbers of homeless people in some areas, there was little hostel or day care provision available.

151   In coastal areas, for example, people were accommodated, out of season, in bed and breakfast accommodation which required residents to leave early in the morning and not to return until the evening. This also occurs in direct-access accommodation.

152   Consequently, day care facilities are a priority requirement.

153   In cities where there is little or no day care provision, and the majority of homeless people are accommodated in bed and breakfast accommodation, obtaining a hot meal presents problems. Soup runs and soup kitchens may provide the only food. Users felt that these were not completely reliable as they did not always turn up, and soup on its own did not offer an adequate or balanced diet.

154   In areas where day care facilities were provided, these services appeared to offer the best chance of access to general mental health services. Day centres became a focal point for the provision of health care services by GPs, psychiatric and general nurses and drug and/or alcohol workers, and welfare rights and housing advisers. They also provided laundry and shower facilities, and a hot meal. These services were more likely to exist in areas in which liaison between the voluntary and statutory services was well developed. These services appeared most sensitive to the needs of homeless people.

*"No job, no home - no home, no job."*

*"The drop-ins help the less accessible people."*

*"People need to be involved, they need an everyday life."*

*"A drop-in centre was dealing with major crises, including homelessness...."*

*"The attitude of the staff was excellent. Users felt respected and were treated as equals."*

*"The input and views were valued and put into practice wherever possible."*

*"There was no opportunity for users to have any real say about the service but they valued the access to health care facilities, GP and welfare rights advice."*

*Quotes taken from user visitors' reports*

### The Accessibility and Responsiveness of Statutory Services

155 Homeless people are acutely aware of how they are viewed by society in general. They often meet with hostility and coldness from staff who do not understand their problems. For this reason, approaching services presents a daunting prospect.

156 The depression, apathy and boredom engendered by homelessness makes it very difficult for users to keep appointments. Health care and rigid appointment systems become a low priority when set against concerns over where to sleep, where to eat and what to do with one's day.

157 The most effective help the visiting teams found was offered by peripatetic teams in two locations. These teams were able to respond flexibly to users' needs by being regularly accessible and approachable in places and at times convenient to homeless people. This sometimes meant outreach work on the streets at 5am.

*"The homeless problem is a contact problem. If there's an excuse, they don't get seen."*

*"When you get to the bottom, you can't get out of it, there's no help ..."*

*"If your face don't fit, they're not interested."*

*"The most accessible services were those that were not mental health services."*

158 Repeatedly, users stated that cafés and churches were more supportive than formal health care systems.

### General Practice

159 The visiting teams of users did find areas where GPs were sympathetic to the needs of homeless people. Some GPs offer surgeries in night shelters or day centres, or register homeless people of no fixed abode, using the GP practice address or that of the local FHSA.

160 As many homeless people lead very transient lives, registering with a GP is often difficult, and the practices themselves may experience problems in tracking down notes and obtaining information on the medical history of homeless people who are temporarily registered with them. This is particularly the case in areas of seasonal migration.

161 The expectation of being unacceptable to practice staff, or acute awareness of their shabby, sometimes dirty state, may make some homeless people react offensively to imagined slights or patronising attitudes. Consequently, many GP practices were reluctant to register homeless people.

162 GPs who are sympathetic to the needs of homeless people and willing to offer them a service may find themselves overwhelmed since the majority of their colleagues refuse to take on any such work.

*"Accessing mental health services, particularly in crisis situations, is virtually impossible if the person experiencing the crisis is not registered with a GP."*

*"They regularly met with violence and aggression on the street. Gangs of youths in town for the weekend break find homeless people a soft target."*

*"Another of their concerns was being able to access a GP. No practice would take them because of their 'no fixed abode' status.... in the near future both could be left on the street, seriously injured, and unable to access emergency services."*

*Quotes from user visitor's report*

*"I don't think the training is put in. They don't have time, they don't understand."*

*"GPs are gatekeepers."*

*"After two years I was lucky to get a GP who sent me to the community mental health team."*

*Quotes from users*

### Specialist Mental Health Services

163   With a few notable exceptions, the visiting teams found few areas where the specialist mental health services were responsive to the needs of homeless people who were mentally ill.

164   Only in two of the areas visited are there teams whose express purpose is to ensure the provision of the appropriate care for homeless people who are mentally ill.

165   Even in these areas, services were not tailored to meet specific needs, and people were expected to fit into existing, sometimes inappropriate services and suffer the additional stigmatising label of mental illness.

*"The community mental health team is in the same building as the child health clinic. You have to wait in the foyer..... It's embarrassing and degrading, especially when your name is called...."*

*"People don't want to be seen at CMHT offices. They don't think of themselves as mentally ill and don't want other people to."*

*"The presentation of help as a mental health service stops people from using it."*

*"The CMHTs do the easy work. The voluntary sector drop-ins deal with the less acceptable."*

*"The local CMHT is for well-dressed and well-heeled people...."*

*Quotes from users*

*"Don't send your dirty, smelly people to our place...."*

*Quote from nurse in charge of a community day hospital talking to a homelessness worker.*

166   On many psychiatric hospital acute wards, discriminatory attitudes about homeless people prevail and only in a few of the areas visited were links between agencies sufficiently strong to ensure that the Care Programme Approach was effectively implemented for people who were homeless.

167   Few ward-based staff appeared to have comprehensive knowledge of the resources available in the community, and some hospital social work

departments were so fully stretched and short-staffed that they too were often unable to provide adequate support and advice.

168   The fear of having no longer-term (move-on) accommodation available created a reluctance on the part of some mental health services to offer inpatient care to homeless people who were mentally ill. This often meant that homeless people were unable to receive hospital treatment until they became so acutely ill that they required compulsory admission under the Mental Health Act 1983.

*"You come out of hospital worse than before you went in."*

*"When I was in hospital, I just saw a psychiatrist for about twenty minutes a week, sometimes less."*

*"There's very little information on the side-effects of medication."*

*"I'm not going into bloody hospital. If you're homeless, you're not seen as a human being, and they use you as a guinea pig."*

*"Nobody told me I'd get better. I thought I'd be ill for ever."*

*"Staff are not trained to think, but to serve the system."*

*"One psychiatrist said 'We don't really want this sort of person in here, do we'."*

*"My psychiatrist is very good. He's got time and he's understanding. You can tell him what you like."*

*"A large number of homeless people have slipped through various nets."*

*Quotes from users*

## Accident and Emergency Departments

169   As homelessness can cause severe stress, incidents of deliberate self-harm are very common.

170   Homeless people are also vulnerable to attacks and muggings, particularly if they are under the influence of alcohol and/or drugs.

171   Out-of-hours crises, when most social services offices, CMHTs and doctors' surgeries are closed, create the most severe problems for hostel workers. Consequently, the only option is to call the police or send people to accident and emergency departments.

*"Nurses don't like overdoses and don't want to know why."*

*"Not one person asked me 'Why?', not one."*

*"I was in and out eight or nine times with overdoses. No one recognised I had problems."*

*"I was left waiting for two and a half hours, vomiting blood in casualty after I took an overdose."*

*Quote from users*

## People with Challenging Behaviour

*"People with so-called personality disorders are frequently dropped by the services. The label is a dustbin label used as a write-off."*

*Quote from user*

172  Visiting teams were frequently confronted with the issue of the problem caused to hostel workers, and fellow users, by those people diagnosed as suffering a personality disorder.

173  Many of this particular group become homeless because of their anti-social behaviour, and hostel and day centre staff felt that they received little support from health care agencies, which appeared to them to consider people, thus diagnosed, as untreatable.

174  It was felt further that the decrease in bed numbers available in psychiatric inpatient units had narrowed the criteria for admission.

*"Ten years ago people with these problems would have been admitted. Now they are too disruptive, taking up staff time and upsetting other patients."*

*Quote from a consultant psychiatrist*

### Housing

*"Over-riding cause of homelessness - the shortage of affordable, appropriate and secure rented accommodation."*

*Quote from an officer of a former Regional Health Authority*

175  Some areas visited had created alliances between the social services and housing departments or had housing forums in operation to determine the accommodation needs of people leaving hospital. These forums consisted of mental health workers, voluntary workers and users.

176  In some areas, housing departments/homeless persons' units were sympathetic to the needs of homeless people and were more flexible in their interpretation of housing legislation.

177  More thought needs to be given to accommodating users. Independent living may not be appropriate when they lack support and have few life-skills.

*"It is no good putting people straight into long-term accommodation. They will only blow it. They need help in general living skills first in a supervised move-on place."*

*"Young people with an assured tenancy will still need support for 12 to 18 months."*

*"You have to go where they put you - away from your friends...."*

*"All my friends came round and started dossing on the floor. They ripped off the tele and the fridge and I lost the flat - I hated living alone."*

*"There's a real need for support to prevent deterioration of flats and loss of deposits."*

*Quotes from users*

*"Users' views have been sought; they must be used constructively."*

*Quote taken from NHS Booklet - Involving local people - Examples of good practice.*

*The General Principles of Good Practice in Commissioning and Delivering Mental Health Services for Homeless People*

# CHAPTER 9

The General Principles
of Good Practice in
Commissioning and
Delivering Mental
Health Services for
Homeless People

## INTRODUCTION

THE GENERAL PRINCIPLES
OF GOOD PRACTICE IN
COMMISSIONING AND
DELIVERING MENTAL
HEALTH SERVICES FOR
HOMELESS PEOPLE

178 A number of reports have highlighted the problems of, and potential solutions to, providing health and social services for homeless mentally ill people. These accounts tend to be descriptive rather than critical evaluations of current provision. The proliferation of studies of the nature and extent of mental health problems among different sub-groups of homeless people (particularly with regard to the characteristics of male hostel residents), has not stimulated the same level of operational research on how to provide effective services for this population. However, what does emerge is that there is no single service solution applicable to all situations. This chapter identifies some of the key components of services for homeless mentally ill people and concludes by looking at the principles underlying good service provision for this generally deprived group.

## EARLIER EXPERIENCES OF DEVELOPING SERVICES FOR HOMELESS MENTALLY ILL PEOPLE IN ENGLAND AND WALES.

179 There have been comparatively few mental health services targeted specifically at homeless mentally ill people in England and Wales.

180 In 1984, the Manchester and Salford Health Care for Homeless People Project was established with two full-time community psychiatric nurses. This service found that the overwhelming majority of homeless people who were referred to it were receiving little or no support from mainstream services.

181 The community psychiatric nurses were therefore involved in clinical work as well as in trying to maintain any existing sources of psychiatric intervention, offering hostel staff support and training about mental health issues, and facilitating communication between the health services and hostel workers.

182 In 1987, a multi-disciplinary psychiatric team was set up in South London to serve four large hostels for homeless men who had a high prevalence of schizophrenia. The team compared a case-management model of service with an assessment and referral service, finding that case-management produced a significantly increased rate of re-housing and a better level of enduring engagement with services. A visiting psychiatric service for hostels has also been reported from Nottingham.

183 In 1989, a mainstream community psychiatric nursing service documented its contacts with homeless clients, finding a high rate of referral from voluntary agencies. It recommended a multi-disciplinary approach.

*"The people who run the drop-in know how to do it."*

184 The current Central London Homeless Initiative established a number of multi-disciplinary teams to provide services for homeless mentally ill people across a range of inadequate accommodations, from the street to squats and hostels. Early data from the evaluation team suggests that large numbers of people referred have severe mental illness and little or no meaningful contact with mainstream psychiatric services. The teams differed in the detail of their organisation and focus; some had a medical, and some had a social work orientation. These appeared to be converging with time. This model of service seems to have addressed the issue of access but its effectiveness remains to be demonstrated. (The evaluation was carried out by Research and Development in Psychiatry - now the Sainsbury Centre).

185    It should be stressed that this is not a finite list of initiatives, and that those
       cited here are simply relevant examples.

## THE PROBLEMS OF PROVIDING SERVICES FOR HOMELESS MENTALLY ILL PEOPLE IN THE UK

*"The homelessness problem is a contact problem. If there's an excuse they won't get seen."*

*Quote from user*

186    Homeless people tend not only to be in poorer health, but also to have
       greater difficulties in gaining access to services when compared to the rest
       of the population.

187    Recent research suggests that about 60% of homeless people do not know
       where to seek help or advice on health or social services related matters
       (Stark et al, 1989). Few had access to appropriate health care and less than
       30% were claiming appropriate benefits or financial support (Stark et al,
       1989; Weller et al, 1987).

### Problems of Registration with a General Practitioner

188    Surveys have illustrated the finding that homeless people are less likely to be
       registered with a GP than the rest of the population.

- In one survey of people living on the streets, under a third were
  registered.

- The registration rate of people living in large direct access hostels was
  found to be similar, although some of these people were registered
  with a GP in their own locality (Stern R, and Stilwell B, 1989 - Margins to
  the Mainstream).

- Detailed surveys of the homeless population in two London Boroughs,
  conducted in 1992 and 1993, showed the average registration rate was
  74% in Hackney and 85% in Newham. Research indicates that the rate
  of registration of the various sub-groups of homeless people was
  directly correlated with the place of each person on the continuum of
  homelessness. In other words, people were least likely to be registered
  if sleeping out or squatting (Hinton, 1993).

*"Provision for homeless people with drug problems was more problematic, largely because this group tends to be younger with more chaotic life-styles."*

- A survey commissioned by an FHSA in the South West of England
  showed that 27% of general practices would fully register a homeless
  person who asked to do so at the practice, 33% would treat
  homeless people as temporary residents, and 24% would offer them
  immediate care if necessary. Only 4% of the fundholding practices
  surveyed reported that they would fully register homeless patients,
  whereas 55% of inner-city practices reported fully registering these
  people. About eight out of 10 of the doctors said that such patients
  were more difficult to treat than other patients. The most frequent
  problems associated with registering homeless people were
  regarded to be their associated social problems (90% agreed), the
  lack of medical records (88% agreed), their complex health problems
  (79% agreed) and associated alcohol or substance misuse (78%
  agreed). The specialist primary health care project team and the
  FHSA were most often perceived as the agencies which should take
  the lead in helping homeless people gain access to specialist health
  care services. Forms of support most frequently requested by GPs
  were a homeless advice centre (81%) and greater knowledge of local
  support groups (57%).

- The length of time a person has been in the UK also has a direct
  correlation to the likelihood of their being registered (Hinton 1993).

- The rate of registration for homeless families has been found to be above 90%.

189 The reasons for low levels of registration are varied.

- Homeless people often view their health as a low priority until a problem becomes a crisis, which then necessitates a visit to an accident and emergency department.

- Homeless people fear the discrimination they may encounter in trying to register with a GP and some report having had bad experiences of contact with the health services in the past.

- High mobility will often mean that someone is a long way from his or her GP when a visit to the surgery is required.

- Homeless people, especially families, may be reluctant to change their GP when they are moved to a new area as they generally aim to return to their home area as soon as possible.

190 Some of the reasons for GPs' reluctance to register homeless people have already been mentioned. Additionally, there may be a misconception that a permanent address is required or concern that homeless persons will not meet the targets for immunisation, screening and health promotion as they may be harder to reach.

191 There is a strong financial disincentive for GPs fully to register homeless patients who end up staying with the practice for less than three months. Current FHSA Red Book guidelines result in practices receiving no payment for these patients.

192 The HAS has come to the opinion that the problem could be, at least partially, resolved if general practices were to receive some payment for fully registering homeless people who stay in a practice area for less than three months. GPs should also receive item-of-service payments for patients who are temporarily registered for cervical cytology and immunisation.

193 GP registration is only one of the problems which affect access to health care since homeless people face other difficulties in gaining access to the full range of health services. A survey in West Lambeth found that even those homeless people who were registered with a GP still used their services less than the rest of their patients, despite their suffering poorer health. Homeless people are more likely to use an accident and emergency department, either to meet primary care needs or to address problems that could have been dealt with by a GP at an earlier stage.

194 In a survey of GP practices in one area visited by the HAS, it was revealed that only about one-quarter of the practices would fully register a homeless person seeking treatment. Very few (4%) of the fundholding practices would do so. This appears to be related to concerns, which were frequently expressed, about the lack of medical records, and the social, mental health and alcohol and substance misuse problems such patients bring. In addition, a number of GPs volunteered the comment that full registration implied an obligation to visit and follow-up patients. This is regarded as a particularly difficult task with regard to some homeless patients. Others mentioned the effect on contract targets - approximately six of 10 GPs expressed this as a concern. There is, therefore, a case which can be made for providing some incentives for GPs to register homeless people, without affecting their contract targets.

195  A much higher percentage of practices located within inner city areas (56%) were prepared to fully register homeless patients. Perhaps, this is because homeless people present themselves more often in inner city areas and the resulting familiarity can lead to greater acceptance by the practices involved. In this context, it is also interesting that significantly fewer of the inner city practices agreed that there was a difficulty in referring homeless patients to secondary services.

196  This evidence is at variance with that for homeless families. A survey of people living in temporary accommodation in the former North West Thames Region showed substantially higher rates of consultation with GPs and of visiting accident and emergency departments compared to those of the resident population (Victor, 1992).

197  Poor use of primary care leads to a correspondingly higher level use of secondary care services. Research, conducted by the King's Fund, discovered that homeless people were far more likely to have an unplanned admission for acute care than other people in an inner city area. A high proportion of these admissions was to mental health services. Members of homeless families were found to be 2.4 times as likely to have an unplanned acute admission, while research in London showed that the rate for people living on the streets was as high as 4.7 times the average.

*"We've got to have a place to go."*

*Quote from user*

198  Homeless mentally ill people also tend to stay in acute mental illness beds longer than the rest of the population. In one inner London district, up to half the acute mental illness beds were occupied by homeless people.

## TOWARDS GOOD PRACTICE

199  Before detailing the key principles of good practice, it is useful to review the debate on special versus mainstream mental health services for homeless people which surfaced in the service visits made by the HAS (chapter 7).

### Special or Mainstream Mental Health Service Provision?

200  It is clear that some mental health services have failed to offer access to key groups of people who are most in need of their support. There is less agreement about how services should respond. A debate continues about whether it is better to set up a special service, exclusively for homeless people, or to improve the full range of services to ensure they are sensitive and responsive to the needs of all who require them, including people who are homeless.

201  Special services have often been developed by committed individuals frustrated by the failure of mainstream services to treat homeless people. These special services ensure that homeless people can gain access to the care they need but there are risks that these services could prove less comprehensive than mainstream services. In the short-term, the special service approach meets a demand for action, but it may, in turn, undermine pressure for lasting change in the rest of the local mental health and local authority services. By offering a clear focus for care, which homeless people know how to use, a special service can also provide a rationale for other services to exclude homeless people from them. For instance, there is some evidence that it is not uncommon for local GPs or specialist mental health services to redirect homeless people to the new special services, where they exist. This suggests that the special service approach can, paradoxically, make mainstream services more inaccessible.

202 Increasingly, special services have attempted to ensure that their users are re-integrated into mainstream services. The initiatives taken have included creating mechanisms for registering people with local GPs. This process has often proved difficult to manage, especially at the clinical level where practitioners are involved in engaging users and gaining their trust, only to ask them to move to a different service.

203 In practice, the distinctions between special and mainstream services are often blurred. Often the best method for service development is that of improving both aspects of provision at the same time. Special services offer opportunities for innovation and they ensure that homeless people are not forgotten. They may also serve as sources of expertise to inform and train the staff of other local services and, thereby, improve their provision. The important point, learned from experience, is that the roles for special services should be clearly pinpointed and agreed as should their integration with mainstream services.

## THE KEY PRINCIPLES OF GOOD PRACTICE

204 These key principles of good practice are drawn from the findings of the service visits made by the HAS. They also borrow from the good practice paper *Community Mental Health Services for Homeless People* produced by Access to Health. However, it should be noted that the principles outlined are applicable to any mental health service whether a special one for homeless people or a mainstream service to an entire community. (The key principles are indicated in italics).

*Services should be offered on a drop-in basis with no appointment needed and users should be able to refer themselves and be seen the same day if the need is urgent.*

205 People who are homeless and have mental health problems often find it hard to keep appointments and fit in with systems. So, services should be flexible and be capable of adaptation to users' needs rather than demand that they make adjustments to fit in with services. Services should have a welcoming and non-institutional atmosphere to help people not to feel stigmatised for using them.

*An advocacy role should be central to services offered to homeless people with mental health problems and illnesses.*

206 Lack of housing, poverty and benefit problems, isolation and loneliness, and physical health problems can all be elements contributing to a person's mental health problems. Services should take a broad view of users' needs and try to assist with a range of issues in addition to mental health problems. They should have the capacity for liaison with and referral to workers outside mental health services where necessary. Liaison with housing agencies and homeless persons' units is crucial. Some of the most effective services seen during the visits were those which played a co-ordinating role through work with hostels and day centres and with the health services, and which facilitated access for users to a range of other services.

### The NHS and local authorities should work in partnership with the voluntary sector and with community groups and support the services that people use.

*"There's no user on the housing forum."*

*"The community mental health team is not present at the planning meetings, neither is the housing association."*

207 Traditional mainstream mental health services may not be equipped to provide the services homeless people want in settings which they are willing to visit. It was noted that some people with the highest support needs were not in touch with statutory services at all but were using homelessness drop-ins, unemployed peoples' centres, churches, women's groups, refugee groups, and cafés, to get the support they needed. This must be recognised by the statutory sector and consideration should be given to diverting funding to the places in the community that people with mental health problems do use, and to user groups, to lead their own services.

### Mental health services should put more emphasis on talking and listening.

208 It was often the experience of users that they felt that their community psychiatric nurse only had time to give them an injection or that their GP had no time to listen to them. Users who had taken a number of overdoses felt that the response of the accident and emergency department was a purely medical one and that nobody gave them time to talk. It should be recognised, particularly when working with homeless people, that they need time to talk and that building trust is slow work. Clinical staff, who work with homeless people, should have this need for extra time acknowledged and reflected in the size of their case loads. Additionally, monitoring processes should acknowledge the time commitments of staff working with homeless people when evaluating outcomes.

### Community mental health services should be publicised effectively with their potential users.

*"Most people rely on word of mouth to hear about services. "*

*"There is a lack of advice on complementary therapies and counselling."*

*Quotes from users*

209 Publishing the existence and work of community health services should be carried out through the voluntary organisations and community groups which work with homeless people and by distributing information at sites where homeless people gather. Information should be appropriate and relevant to the lives of people who are homeless.

### The services should provide high quality clinical expertise, and evaluation of their effectiveness should be an integral part of the work.

*"Staff are not trained to think but to serve the system."*

*Quote from user*

210 Skilled and experienced staff should be recruited to mental health services. Their expertise may be used by many groups and organisations through their involvement in teaching programmes for staff of various disciplines and in speaking at workshops and conferences. Some of the prime roles of specialist services are those of education, training, advice, liaison, consultation and co-ordination with other more general services.

211 Evaluation is an important part of the work of all services. Data on client contacts, interventions and outcomes should be systematically gathered and reports produced regularly.

***It is important that work should be carried out across agency boundaries and services should, where possible, be jointly commissioned.***

212 Services are more likely to respond effectively to the multiple needs of homeless people with mental health problems if they are based on a multi-agency approach at the commissioning level and at the level of service provision to individual clients. For example, panels made up of representatives from the health service and the social services and housing departments could match individuals and their needs to the housing options available. They could also plan support packages to carry out the duties of the statutory services for vulnerable people. These duties are contained in the legislation relating to homelessness.

***A diverse client group requires diverse services.***

213 It should not be assumed that people with mental health problems, or that homeless people, are homogeneous groups. Homeless people with mental health problems include women, young people, elderly people, people with distinct language and cultural needs, gay men and lesbians. The provision of services should be sensitive to the needs of these different groups and ensure that they do not feel excluded.

***Outreach work and out-of-hours services are appropriate and important responses to the needs of this client group.***

214 Many of the teams serving homeless mentally ill people, met by the HAS during its visits, had tried to conduct outreach work in a variety of non-traditional ways. Locations included night shelters, bed and breakfast hotels and street doorways and work, sometimes with workers from other voluntary organisations that actively seek people who may need their services.

215 Approaching people when working away from a base or other support demands particular skills. Contacts with very damaged and disadvantaged users require time to be taken to build trusting relationships, assess the complex needs of the clients/patients and then help them to gain access to the support and treatment they need. Selection of staff who are able to take this sensitive approach is a key issue. Services that are available in the evenings and at weekends, when homeless people are particularly likely to experience crises, are also important considerations. It is important to stress the need for continuity of contact between particular outreach workers and individual clients.

*"These people are normal, why treat them like freaks?"*

*"We don't want to sit down, smoke and drink tea all the time."*

*Quotes from user*

216 These principles and elements of good practice are summarised in Table 4.

*Table 4*

| **Elements of Good Practice in Providing Community Mental Health Services for Homeless People** |
| --- |
| • Drop-in services with self referral. |
| • Liaison and advocacy roles emphasise the requirement for an holistic approach to service commissioning and provision. |
| • Work in partnership with voluntary and community groups. |
| • Emphasis on listening - services and their staff should be perceived by users as welcoming and approachable. |
| • Effective information and publicity. |
| • Multi-agency working. |
| • High quality clinical expertise with built-in evaluation. |
| • Outreach work and out-of-hours services. |

*"The most accessible services are those that are not mental health services."*

*Quote from user visitor report*

217  As this document highlights, homeless people are likely to present complex combinations of psychological, social and physical problems. These difficulties can be organised into a hierarchy of need, but for most homeless people their basic requirements, especially for housing, take precedence over the acquisition of treatment for mental illness. Engaging homeless people in services, therefore requires providers to remedy any mismatch between the users' expectations and their own. It is important to be prepared to negotiate the order of priorities flexibly in order to ensure that engagement with services is not a major obstacle.

*"You need to be in a fit state to know your rights."*

*"I want some proper, structured counselling."*

*"The nurses haven't got time."*

*"One, a night nurse, was really good. She talked to me and really understood."*

*"Do they know their jobs? Do they help you? Do they hell!"*

*Quotes from users*

218  Most services for homeless mentally ill people acknowledge the importance of multi-disciplinary team work and the use of case management. The latter may be particularly important in helping to negotiate the bureaucratic and practical hurdles encountered when trying to gain access to health and social care and support. Studies have found that only one-third of homeless mentally ill people know how or where to obtain help with their housing, financial, social, or health needs (Scott, 1992).

219  Finally, a major issue that should be addressed is the problem of the negative attitudes towards homeless mentally ill people expressed by many professionals. Mentally ill people are a stigmatized group within society, but homeless mentally ill people are at risk of being doubly disadvantaged if they encounter such attitudes from the professions. This report attempts to offer some insights into the complex field of homelessness and sees training and inter-agency working as the key means of changing negative attitudes.

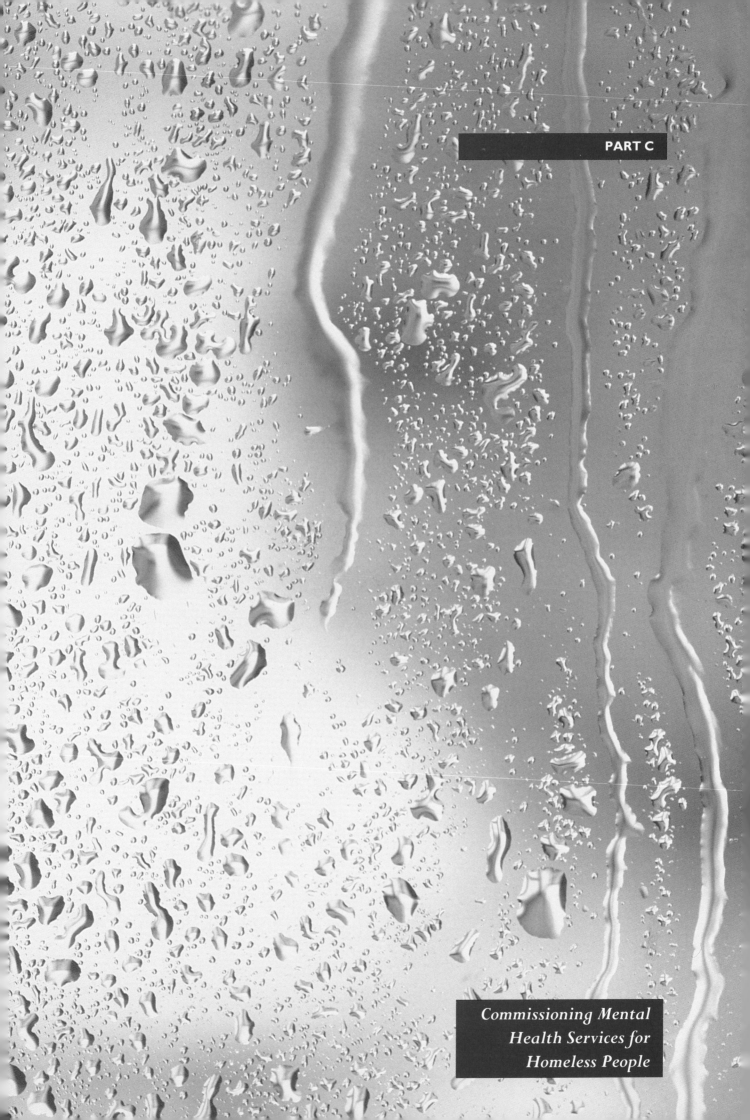

**PART C**

*Commissioning Mental Health Services for Homeless People*

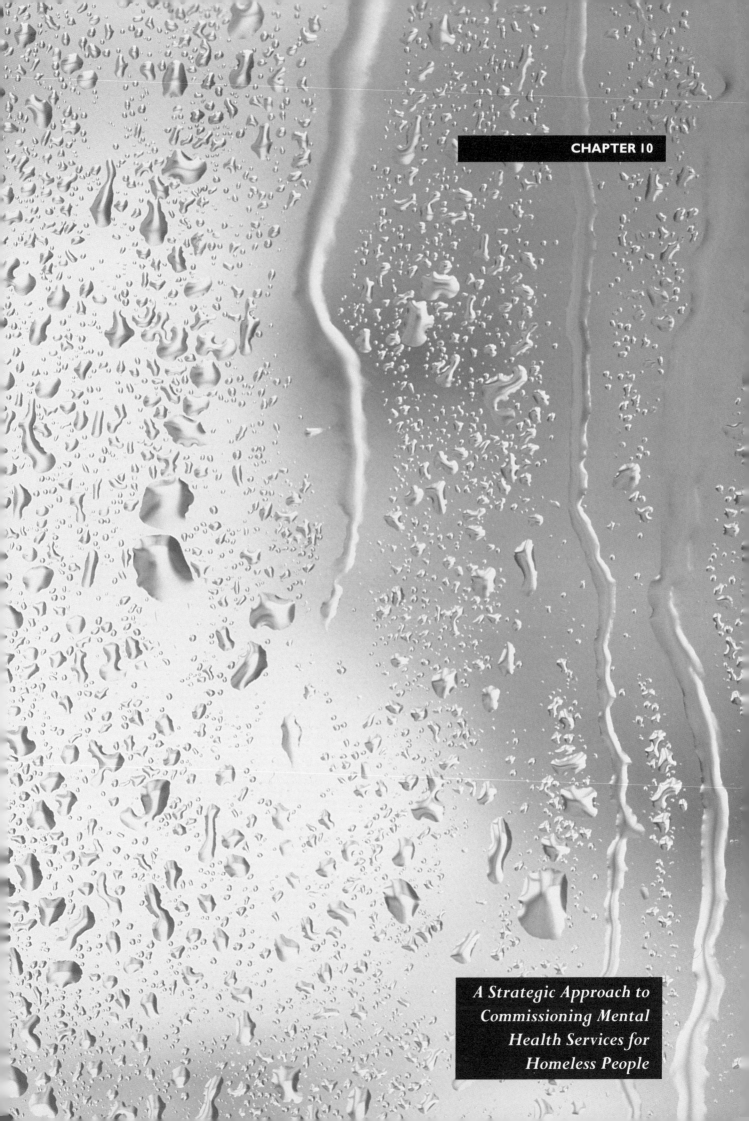

**CHAPTER 10**

*A Strategic Approach to Commissioning Mental Health Services for Homeless People*

## INTRODUCTION

220 The further development of commissioning and purchasing in the broadest sense is a key task for the NHS. In this context, the view of the HAS is that examination of the commissioning and delivery of services for homeless mentally ill people is a key means of testing current performance by purchasers and providers. Evidence from the service visits suggests that a service which is accessible to this highly deprived client group is likely to be generally responsive to the needs of the mentally ill people as a whole. Also, examination of purchaser and provider performance in this area can be a good qualitative test of delivery of mental health services generally.

221 This section of the report focuses particularly on commissioning and has been structured around the model of good practice set out in *Purchasing for Health* (1993).

222 The NHS Executive, in 1993, defined three key goals for purchasers who should buy to:

- improve people's health by targeting resources on effective ways of delivering clinical care and promoting health;

- improve the quality of health care, making it more responsive to the wishes and needs of people; and

- ensure that as many people as possible receive high quality care from what available resources can provide.

223 *Purchasing for Health* sets out *seven stepping stones*. The service visits highlighted good practice and this, in turn, supports the seven key areas for purchaser performance identified in *Purchasing for Health*. The areas were:

- Strategy

- Improving the knowledge base of purchasing

- Effective contracts

- Increasing responsiveness to local people

- Development of mature relations with providers

- Developing local alliances

- Improving the organisational capacity of purchasers

This review will look at each of these areas in turn with specific reference to homeless people.

224 As well as identifying the areas noted above, the guidance in *Purchasing for Health* outlines seven imperatives for effective contracting. These will be considered in detail later as part of the discussion of current practice and performance.

225 The rest of this section covers the key areas noted above and draws on the findings from the service visits and the more general examination of good practice undertaken as part of this thematic review.

A STRATEGIC APPROACH
TO COMMISSIONING
MENTAL HEALTH
SERVICES FOR HOMELESS
PEOPLE

*"In a nutshell, its money."*

Quote from user

## STRATEGY

### Awareness and Models of Commissioning

226　A critical question arising from both the fieldwork component of this review and from a survey of published strategies is the one of awareness of homelessness and mental health as an issue at all. In 1993, the HAS established its Library of Commissioning Documentation. Analysis of the contents, provided by 88% of health authorities and commissions in England and Wales, showed that in 1993-94 only 6% mentioned homelessness in their strategies for mental health services. If access to mainstream mental health services for this particularly disadvantaged group is part of strategy, it is more likely that the services will be accessible to all users. *Mental Illness - a Strategy for Wales* (Welsh Office 1989) and the later *Protocol for Investment in Health Gain - Mental Health* from the Welsh Health Planning Forum (1993) have helped to ensure that individual commissioning bodies in Wales are significantly ahead in developing their own strategies.

227　Of the 10 health authorities visited by HAS teams, only two specifically mentioned homelessness and mental illness, although five of the authorities had included homelessness more generally as an area of concern. This was usually considered in the context of enabling access to primary and secondary care services.

*"The negative effects of homelessness on the physical and mental health of homeless people has been recognised for many years."*

*Quote from user visitor report*

228　Homeless people are to be found everywhere, so homelessness needs to be given a specific place in any health strategy. The long-term aim of the strategy should be that of ensuring that homeless people have as full and equal access to mainstream mental health care, and to all other forms of primary and secondary care, as does the domiciled population. It may well be, however, that the pathway to this goal lies in the provision of specially designated services for homeless people in the short-term. This may have the advantages of first, providing a speedy and relevant response to need; second, gaining further knowledge of the problems of access and the distinguishing characteristics of the client group; and third, providing models of service which can be implemented within mainstream services. The decision to develop a short-term approach while a different long-term one is worked-up is a matter for local choice. This should be influenced by the overall numbers of homeless people in an area, the severity of their problems, and the capacity of existing services to meet their needs; that is, it should be informed by consideration of a comprehensive needs assessment, of health gain issues and of the results of compiling an inventory of local resources (mapping).

229　The process of developing and implementing a strategy is not a single finite one. Rather, it is a series of connecting processes which feed into each other, leading back to review and adjustment over time. The work of the HAS with commissioning mental health services, through its analysis of the contents of the HAS Library of Commissioning Documentation and through study of the more effective commissioners, (Williams, 1994; Williams and Richardson, 1995; Cumella et al, 1995), suggests an idealised approach to commissioning mental health services and this is summarised in Figures 2 and 3. They are applicable to ensuring effective commissioning of mental health services for homeless mentally ill people.

**230** Outline strategy formulation triggers the subsequent activity, going through all the stages of needs assessment, determination of priorities, moving from outline plans for implementation to detailed service specifications, monitoring, evaluation and strategy review.

*Figure 2*

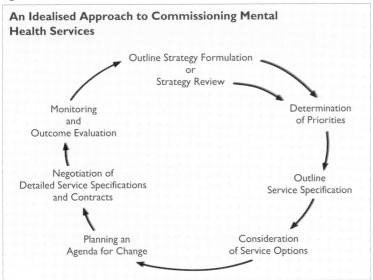

**An Idealised Approach to Commissioning Mental Health Services**

Outline Strategy Formulation
or
Strategy Review

Determination of Priorities

Monitoring and Outcome Evaluation

Negotiation of Detailed Service Specifications and Contracts

Outline Service Specification

Planning an Agenda for Change

Consideration of Service Options

**231** It is important to ensure that everyone concerned operates to agreed criteria and that definitions for recording data and providing services are complementary. In this instance, an example could be the agreement to adopt the definition of homelessness used in the Housing Act 1985.

**232** The route from an outline to more detailed strategy passes through a number of stages. A key issue in this process, which faces all commissioners, is that of determining priorities. Health needs assessment should lead to the exercise of a balanced consideration of the clinical realities, health gain and user and carer opinions. This in turn allows for local goals to be set against awareness of the capabilities and capacities of existing local services (obtained by mapping local resources). This background information should enable priorities for service commissioning, provision and development to be better agreed and identified with providers and partner agencies, and for a more detailed and agreed strategy to be formulated.

*Figure 3*

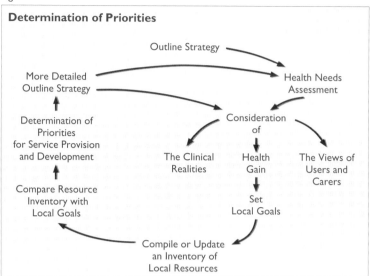

**Determination of Priorities**

233 The goals, objectives and operational tactics for meeting the needs of homeless mentally ill people which can be set by bringing together the concepts of health gain and service targeting spring from a mature strategy. The contents of Table 5 offer suggestions on improving mental health care resulting from an appropriate strategy.

*"No recent survey of the mental health needs of homeless people has been undertaken."*

*Quote from user visitor report*

Table 5

| Improving Mental Health Sevices for Homeless People | |
|---|---|
| HEALTH GAIN AREA | SERVICE TARGETS |
| 1. DEVELOPING ACCESS<br><br>• Increase the number of initial contacts between homeless people and clinicians. | TARGETS<br><br>• Invest in multi-disciplinary outreach work in both primary and mental health care.<br><br>• Involve fundholding and non-fundholding GPs in strategy formulation.<br><br>• Increase the uptake of registration with GPs.<br><br>• Maximise access to GPs via sessional work and outreach surgeries. |
| 2. HEALTH PROMOTION<br><br>• Seek to reduce the incidence of physical and mental ill health problems in homeless people. | TARGETS<br><br>• Thematic information programmes, eg alcohol, depression.<br><br>• Publicity targeted on Health of the Nation objectives.<br><br>• Mobile screening units.<br><br>• Joint clinics with social services, including advice on benefits. |
| 3. CO-ORDINATION<br><br>• Provide a co-ordinated and flexible service which can respond sensitively to the special and complex needs of homeless people. | TARGETS<br><br>• Establish formalised systems and protocols for liaison between relevant agencies and services in respect of this client group. |
| 4. INFORMATION<br><br>• Provide appropriate levels of care based upon assessment of individual need. | TARGETS<br><br>• Develop common systems of information gathering and exchange between relevant agencies, including social services housing and the voluntary sector.<br><br>• Ensure that the Care Programme Approach and other care management and planning processes encompass homeless mentally ill people.<br><br>• Develop collaborative care monitoring systems with other agencies. |
| 5. HOUSING AND RESETTLEMENT<br><br>• Work with appropriate agencies, to ensure provision of short-term, medium-term and permanent accommodation for homeless people. | TARGETS<br><br>• Participate in local and voluntary housing sector planning processes.<br><br>• Collaborate in the establishment of co-ordinating housing bodies such as trusts and consortia.<br><br>• Ensure the local authority exercises its nomination rights to housing association tenancies.<br><br>• Employ, or fund, experienced resettlement workers.<br><br>• Assist the local authority homeless persons unit by input into assessments by ensuring the availability of clinical staff. |

234 The Service Targets and possible Health Gains listed in Table 5 are prompted by the approach of the Welsh Office NHS Directorate's *Protocol for Investment in Health Gain - Mental Health.* The references in that document to homelessness and housing should ensure that these are treated as integral elements in any mental health strategy and that services are promoted which offer sensitive responses to the needs of homeless people.

### Involving GPs in Strategy

235 A key message from the service visits was that of the importance of there being a clear strategy agreed by the purchasers for the major statutory agencies. This was seen as the best way of improving the often fragmentary and ad hoc availability of mental health care to homeless people. The role of GPs in this context is crucially important. As an increasingly significant body of purchasers, fundholding and non-fundholding GPs should be involved from the start in the formulation of any plans to provide primary mental health and specialist mental health services to homeless people. This should be an element in their business plans and seen as particularly important in areas where the majority of the domiciled population is registered with fundholding practices. In these areas, access to primary and secondary health care services will be directly influenced by fundholders' requirements.

236 An aim, agreed between purchasers, should be that full registration with a GP is available to homeless people, as the best means of offering continuity of care and knowledge of the individual. At the same time, access on both a temporary and an 'immediate and necessary' basis is required to primary health care teams. Where homeless people received a high quality service from general practitioners in the areas visited, it was found that there were arrangements in force for sessional GP work which carried additional payments.

### Linking Services in Planning

*"Statutory responsibility for long-term strategic planning needs to be developed. The voluntary sector has dominated needs assessment, provision and planning of services for homeless people, including those with mental health problems."*

Quote from user visitor report

237 A joint strategy which recognises the requirement to provide services for homeless people should be able to suggest ways of avoiding rigid compartmentalisation. Symptoms of mental disorder in this group can often be accompanied by problems of drug and/or alcohol misuse, and by a range of physical health problems. Multi-disciplinary teams, with workers who have a range of skills and experience, offer the possibility of a more holistic approach and greater ease of access for the client group.

238 The agreed strategy should be made public to everyone working in services for homeless people. It should be shared and reviewed with providers at all levels. The HAS service visitors found several places where purchasers had developed sophisticated, coherent strategies which had never been seen by provider middle managers or teams working at the front line. Strategy is the starting point but it is not a static tool. It should be seen as a constant reference point.

### Multi-agency Strategic Planning

239 Planning is a specially complex activity because of the heterogeneous and constantly changing nature of the client groups, in terms of numbers and seasonal flow and the diverse nature of their requirements.

240 An holistic approach should ensure that all the basic requirements are considered. These include the items in Table 6:

*Table 6*

| The Basic Requirements of Homeless People |
| --- |
| • Somewhere to stay |
| • Something to eat |
| • Laundry facilities |
| • Health care |
| • Social care |
| • Access to more permanent housing |
| • Access to training, education and employment |
| • Access to recreation |

*"There should be a better, more modern approach to enabling users to live successfully in the community - a more psycho-holistic approach."*

*Quote from user visitor report*

241 Encompassing all of these means that both service needs and planning assessment for this group is best undertaken on a multi-agency basis involving the core local authority (social services and housing) and health services purchasers, as well as others. These include health and social service providers, police and probation services, education and employment services and, most importantly, voluntary and charitable sector agencies. The last of these may be the largest providers of services specifically orientated to homeless people.

*"There seems to be a major breakdown in communication between various organisations."*

*Quote from user*

*"When you get to the bottom you can't get out, there's no help."*

*Quote from girl living under a bridge, washing her hair in the river and clothes in the toilet*

## Healthy Alliances with Housing Departments and the Voluntary Sector

242 Delivery of services to this client group critically depends on the development of healthy alliances between purchasers and service providers in a range of different sectors. The HAS fieldwork found that some of the most impressively organised services in the health authority areas visited had grown up through development of partnerships often led by the non-statutory or voluntary sectors. Often, a critical partnership was that between social services and housing departments. Where relationships were poor or responsibilities widely distributed, service delivery was more likely to be poor. For example, one of the health authorities visited related to a number of different district councils in respect of housing, two county councils in respect of social services and a number of different mental health providers. In this area, co-ordination of the planning of mental health services had not risen to the challenge represented by this difficult configuration.

*"It's just a business philosophy – there's no humanity."*

*"There's no one with forward-thinking."*

*Quotes from users*

## Involving Service Users

*"User involvement is just tokenistic."*

*Quote from user*

243  In addition to the involvement of statutory and independent agencies in the formulation of strategy, there is a need to actively seek the views of users and potential users in order to commission services which are sensitive to the distinctive needs of homeless people. There is no single formula which guarantees success, and every effort should be made to avoid a token approach. It is also wise to remember that most voluntary agencies' views are not directly representative of service users. Some of the areas visited in the fieldwork had established effective county-wide forums of mental health service users who had a direct input into strategic planning groups. None, however, were identified which included people who were homeless.

*"There needs to be an effective mental health forum involving the statutory services, voluntary sector services and an effective user voice that includes homeless people and black users."*

*Quote from user visitor report*

*Table 7*

| A Checklist of Options for Involving Users |
| --- |
| • Set up consultative planning forums for users, with facilitation provided. |
| • Include at least two service users on regular single-service or joint planning groups. |
| • Appoint skilled advocates to liaise with users and feedback to commissioners. |
| • Undertake interviews with and visits to users. |
| • Ensure that users have the chance to comment on Community Care Plans. |

## Integrating Housing Need into Strategy

*"Staff felt there was a general lack of hostel provision for couples."*

*Quote from user visitor report*

244  In strategic planning for homeless people, there should be a long-term plan for developing a wide range of supported accommodation services, covering direct access beds, high care, minimum care, short-term, and homes for life. These are not the responsibility of a single purchaser. An integrated strategy, which may be followed by joint or 'mirror-image' commissioning, will help to ensure a response which is flexible and comprehensive. It is recognised that where changes in local government result in unitary authorities being established, integration of housing services with strategic planning may be made easier. In any event, resource mapping of housing provision is required, which generates a clear view of the respective roles of the housing association movement and public sector housing developments. It may be that one way forward is to set up an arms-length co-ordinating body such as a housing consortium or separate trust to pull together the strands. This, in itself, will be a strategic decision which will need a clear notion of whether such a body is a purchaser or a provider of services, or covers both functions.

*"The scale of the problems that homeless people (in Central London) were experiencing had forced the government to support organisations that provide high quality, modern, projects for homeless people, by providing funding which enables homeless agencies to do some high quality work, not just in the short-term, but for the foreseeable future."*

*Quote from user visitor report*

## NEEDS ASSESSMENT AND THE KNOWLEDGE-BASE

245 Homeless people have wide and complex health needs, alongside other social needs. Therefore, their use of services may not follow the usual patterns of other users and it is essential that all purchasing authorities take steps to develop and maintain a sound and broad knowledge-base.

246 This must include an assessment of the extent and nature of the health problems of homeless people in their locality. Information should be sought from as many agencies as possible, including health providers, primary health care services, relevant local authority departments, including housing, and the voluntary sector. It may have to be acknowledged that traditional health care services and their associated information systems may not be the best source of this information and that what exists may not be in a readily accessible form or a single location. The voluntary sector may have more up-to-date information, and its long involvement and expertise in this area should be acknowledged. The opinions of other agencies should be used, and any information should be shared on a multi-agency basis.

247 If a health authority is at the initial stages of building its knowledge-base on homelessness, its officers should consider the appropriateness and feasibility of commissioning a specific study to identify the homeless population and their health needs. This would form the basis for development of knowledge in subsequent years. Initiatives of this kind are likely to be particularly beneficial in areas with high homeless populations. Examples of authorities which have conducted this type of research recently include the London Boroughs of Newham and Hackney.

*"Planners will 'listen' to documents far more than to representatives at meetings."*

Quote from user

248 The services from which information could be gained include those listed in Table 8.

*Table 8*

| Information Sources |
| --- |
| • Local authority social services departments |
| • Local authority homeless persons sections |
| • General practitioners |
| • Voluntary organisations that work with homeless people |
| • Voluntary organisations that work with mentally ill people |
| • Health visitors |
| • Census returns |
| • The probation service |
| • Accident and emergency services |
| • Hostels |
| • Night shelters |

249 Local situations are unlikely to be static. Provider services may change in response to changes in priorities and shifts in demand, changes in resources or even changes in clinical interest. These should be monitored constantly. Regular contract reviews should include the capacity to consider the impact of services for vulnerable people who run the risk of being overlooked or excluded from a service.

250 The local population of homeless people may also alter due to seasonal factors, economic and housing changes, and also short and longer-term shifts in population demography.

251 Contracts should be based on a sound knowledge of local health needs and up-to-date awareness of the provider organisations in the locality and their capabilities, in terms not only of quantity but of the quality of their services, including their management. Purchasers need to be aware of the capabilities of providers and this should include their capabilities now and in the future. This should be seen in terms not only of the quantity and capacity of their service, but also of the quality and management capability of the services.

**Establishing a Sound Knowledge-Base**

252 A good knowledge-base should also include general background information about how purchasers and providers in other parts of the country meet the needs of their own homeless people. Examples of best practice elsewhere, which can be adapted to local needs, should be sought. The use of benchmarking with other organisations may foster the development and sharing of good practice. The voluntary sector may well be able to contribute to this process, affecting the delivery, in relationship to quality and access, of services.

In establishing a sound knowledge-base, a key issue is that of *looking to all sources of information.* Examples include the following:

*Data from accident and emergency departments*

- Accident and emergency department attendance records for people of no fixed abode (NFA) housing status.

- The nature and capacity of follow-up services offered to attenders at these departments.

*Care Programme Approach*

- Information from CPA recording systems.

*Housing status, as part of all assessments*

- Does it show equality of access to services?

*Information from homeless units and special services in the locality*

*Notification systems*

- The systems used in Barnet and Tower Hamlets where the homeless persons' unit notifies health providers about the movement of homeless households.

### GP contact data

- Temporary registrations.

- GP services to homeless people.

### Data from local authority housing and social services departments

### Data on local demographic circumstances

- The ethnic mix, age and family structure of the homeless population. (Single parents may be hidden in bed and breakfast houses and single people in temporary housing).

### The needs of the children of homeless people

- Information can be gained from liaison with health visitors.

### Seasonal changes

- Account should be taken of holiday seasons which may result in an influx of temporary visitors and temporary workers in some places.

- Travelling people may also pass through the area in large numbers, or settle for a season. So, there is a need to be aware of population flows within the district.

### The location and nature of services currently provided

- A resource inventory compiled on single agency basis and on the basis of sharing information between sectors of care.

- Issues relating to accessibility, ie locality, opening times, cultural sensitivity.

### The information systems of the provider organisations

- What systems do providers have? Is the data that is collected by them in compatible formats?

- Do the information and contract monitoring systems measure access to and take-up of the services provided?

- Are contracts being effectively delivered?

### The quality and audit systems in existence

- Do any have a specific relevance to, or impact on, the quality of services for homeless people?

### The use of epidemiological data to target services

- Services for children of mothers in bed and breakfast accommodation.

- The use of drug and alcohol misuse services by homeless people.

### Way in which the views of service users are taken into account in monitoring and developing services

*Collection of knowledge on known and effective interventions from elsewhere, and its incorporation into service specifications*

### Other important information

There are other kinds of information that will help to build a sound knowledge-base:

- The training and attitudes of staff towards the problems of homelessness and how they affect service use

  - Are the specific needs of homeless people incorporated in the training for GPs and identified specialist staff?

  - Are there ways of improving service use and satisfaction of clients by staff training and education?

  - Would monitoring systems detect the changes?

- Dissemination of information to service users

  - Are the service users aware of the service contracts?

  - Is the dissemination of this information part of the contract? How do you know?

- Mechanisms for communicating the contents of contracts to all those involved in their delivery

  - Is there a system to monitor communications? How do all the separate players link together?

*Mechanisms for ensuring that the results of information gathering inform future decisions*

253 After all this information has been gathered and agreed, the next steps should include regular contacts with the professionals, managers and workers in the field to establish the most pressing areas of unmet need and areas of least effective service delivery.

## COUNTING HOMELESS PEOPLE

254 Not all those persons who can be categorised as being homeless or at risk of homelessness can be easily identified and counted to enable a quantitative assessment of need.

255 However, official figures are available for people falling into five main accommodation types. Although these are an underestimate, they should enable a base-line estimation of local homelessness to be determined. The categories of homelessness for which figures are available are as follows:

- Temporary accommodation

- Squatting

- Hostels

- Sleeping-out

- Travellers

256 It should be remembered that this method of counting is extremely rough and results in the minimum number of homeless people in these categories. Purchasers in most areas will find that they need to do additional work in order to consider specific matters relating to their homeless population.

## Temporary Accommodation

257    There are people who have been accepted as being statutorily homeless by a local authority under the Housing Act 1985. They may first be housed in bed and breakfast hotels, in property rented from the private sector - a practice known as private sector leasing (PSL) - or in hostels. Some people are classed as being homeless at home, meaning that they are living in accommodation which has been assessed as unsuitable for them, until they can be rehoused.

258    In discharging their legal obligations to house people, local authorities must keep records of the numbers they accept as homeless and make quarterly returns to the Department of the Environment (DoE). These figures can be obtained from the DoE or direct from the council concerned.

259    The temporary accommodation figures required by the DoE are broken down into four categories by dwelling place:

-    bed and breakfast;

-    hostels (including womens' refuges);

-    others (including leased and short-life dwellings); and

-    homeless at home awaiting permanent accommodation.

260    Adding together the figures from these four categories will give a total of homeless households in temporary accommodation. Multiplying the resulting figure by a factor of 2.4 (the average size of homeless households according to a survey by the London Housing Unit and the London Research Centre) will give a rough estimate of the number of individuals in temporary accommodation.

261    Where a health authority has coterminous boundaries with a local authority, the homelessness figures of the council will be directly applicable to the health authority, assuming that the council places its homeless people within its own boundaries. However, this latter circumstance is frequently not the case, especially in London and some other metropolitan boroughs. Where there are no coterminous boundaries, analysis can be undertaken at a local authority ward level, as wards are less likely to be split between DHAs.

## Squatting

262    Boroughs and district councils make an annual return to the DoE, through their Housing Investment Programmes (HIP), of the number of their properties which are in unlicensed occupation - in other words, squatted. This figure only gives part of the picture since not all squatters occupy council property.

263    The Advisory Service for Squatters recorded the ownership of over 2,000 squats in 1991 and found that 26% of squatters were not in local authority property. The 26% of the total number of squatters not in council dwellings constitute a number equal to 35% of those who are in local authority property. So, adding 35% to the DoE figure gives a good estimate for the number of squatters in an area, although local prevalence of squatting may need investigation to fine-tune local projections.

264 A multiplying factor of three should be used to convert numbers of households to numbers of individuals.

## Hostels

*"I suppose they think we are dirty so we only deserve dirty surroundings."*

*"Homeless hostels have stairs, no gardens, no facilities for children, shared kitchens, and rubbish bags thrown out of windows or left in corridors to stink."*

*"This hostel is filthy dirty, it stinks and it's dangerous, it's a fire hazard."*

*Quotes from users*

265 Hostels are of many different types and the definition of a hostel for needs analysis should include emergency night shelters, short-stay hostels and traditional hostels (common lodging houses). This will exclude hostel-dwellers in supported accommodation for people with mental health problems, ex-offenders, and other groups who may be described as homeless.

266 It is reasonable to reach a figure for hostel dwellers by counting bed spaces. Unfortunately, these figures are only readily available in London. Elsewhere, health authorities will need to contact agencies working with homeless people to gain estimates of hostel bed spaces. These will be largely in the voluntary or commercial sectors, but may include the public sector where local authorities provide directly for homeless people.

## Sleeping Out

267 People who sleep out are the most difficult to count. The most up-to-date figures available are contained in the 1991 Census Supplementary Monitor on People Sleeping Rough. As the OPCS advises, poor weather on census night may have affected the numbers who slept out and the count will have missed people who sleep out from time to time. People who sleep out may also deliberately hide themselves for reasons of personal security, and this is another factor which makes them hard to count.

268 The Supplementary Monitor lists numbers by local authority and this raises problems where council and health authorities do not have coterminous boundaries. However, the locations of the wards where people were counted can be obtained from OPCS and this should enable health authorities to gauge more accurately the populations for which they are responsible.

269 Accurate data on those sleeping out will be dependent on regular local surveying of this population and can be supplemented by data collected on service contacts. Again, voluntary agencies working with homeless people often have useful information on numbers and places where rough sleepers can be found.

## Travellers

270 Twice a year, local authorities count the number of gipsy caravans in their local area in which people are living and those figures are collated by the DoE. Three categories are recorded: unauthorised, council, and private encampments. The 2.4 factor of multiplication used for households in temporary accommodation can be used to give a total of individuals living in caravans.

271 Data collected in this way will be more comprehensive than that available now in most areas but it is still likely to underestimate the numbers of caravan dwellers and thus it should be supplemented by local sampling. Further, not all travellers live in caravans and, in rural areas, where the homelessness figures may be small, some people may live in 'benders' or other roughly made forms of shelter.

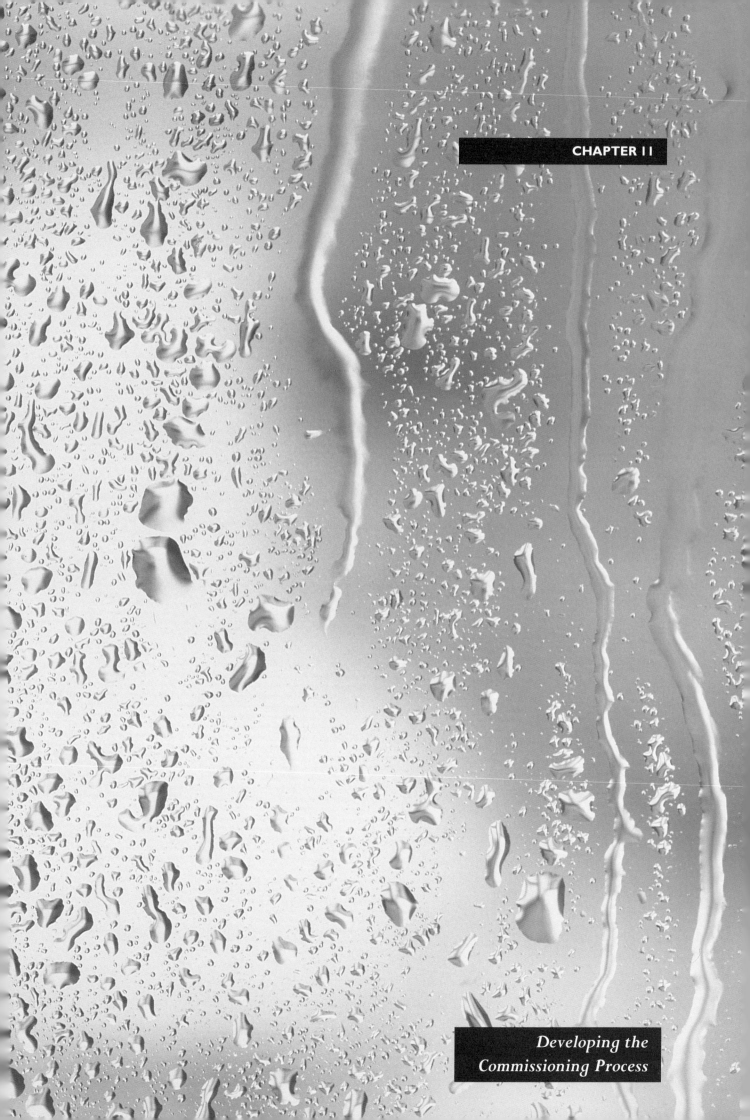

**CHAPTER 11**

*Developing the
Commissioning Process*

## ORGANISATIONAL CAPACITY

**272** In *Purchasing for Health - A Framework for Action (1993)*, the need to strengthen the managerial and professional expertise of purchasers was highlighted as a major element in ensuring that the other aspects of the agenda set by *Purchasing for Health* could be met. These challenges relate to:

- purchasers' knowledge-base; and

- their organisational capacity to deliver appropriate health care to the population through the contracting process.

**273** Purchasing services for homeless mentally ill people is an especially challenging part of the task, as it tests organisational capacity to the limits. Some of the reasons are as follows:

- In order to achieve an acceptable service, purchasers need to understand and devise ways of meeting the needs of 'hard to reach' sections of the community they serve. Homeless people are an obvious example of this category, and thus they pose a significant test of the ability to provide a responsive service. It is complicated by the differing statutory responsibilities (which do not mesh) of the health, social services and housing authorities.

- If they fail in this respect, some services may continue to be inappropriately used, and others underused and ineffectual, or fail to recognise the particular needs of homeless people who are mentally ill. Purchasers may need to invest in training on these issues, for their own staff and also ensure that health, and voluntary providing bodies include relevant training in the continuing professional development. The training needs of primary health care teams should be remembered.

- As the size of this local authority client group is difficult to measure, and heterogeneous in character, demands for services are not likely to be constant, either geographically or over time. However, the group is also highly deprived, and, on any category of need, would be a prime target for intervention by purchasers. This applies even when the overall number of people involved is small, as in some rural areas. This may require the development of locally specific networks for the collection of information in conjunction with other providing agencies to inform all stages in the commissioning process.

- A secondary test of commissioning organisational capacity is the purchaser's ability to correlate information and contacts with appropriate providers in endeavouring to meet the identified needs of the client group.

- A further key organisational objective is that of ensuring that the purchasing agency has a clear strategy for multi-agency co-operation in all stages of the commissioning process.

## KEY ORGANISATIONAL ISSUES

**274** The fieldwork and research undertaken as part of this review identified a number of key issues relating to organisational capacity. The most important of these are set out here.

- There is evidence that the most effective services are provided where there is strong networking across agency boundaries. For example, in one area, the HAS found that good liaison between health, social and housing services ensured that an appropriate range of move-on accommodation for homeless mentally ill people was available.

- Housing departments are essential partners if access to good housing provision (both local authority and housing association stock) is to be achieved. Involvement of housing authorities in consultation in the commissioning process helps to ensure that the Housing Act 1985 is interpreted in a sufficiently flexible way as to better meet the housing needs of homeless mentally ill people.

- Purchasers should be aware that the operation of effective individual care programmes is only possible with strong inter-agency co-operation. Joint working ensures that care programmes are tailored to meet individual need, and this is particularly so if voluntary agencies are integrated into the process alongside hospital and other community-based mental health services. The HAS found that this was aided by training arranged jointly and across agency boundaries as well as by cross-sectoral work to share the work of defining and identifying needs.

- Creating a clear strategy for multi-agency co-operation is a primary test of high level management skills. Where investment is to be made in a particular service, there should be a high degree of clarity about the purpose of that service. (This may seem self-evident, but HAS visiting teams found a lack of clarity or cross-agency agreement about the purpose of high cost services, such as day hospitals, in a number of areas.)

- Targets should be set to be incremental. Rolling contracts may be beneficial as they can be introduced to allow for adaptation as requirements change. A developmental approach to task management in both purchaser and provider organisations is important in supporting endeavours to meet the needs of this client group.

- If appropriate and effective systems are to be delivered, more sophisticated (and cost-effective) monitoring systems need to be developed to ensure that this 'hard to reach' client group is not only able to gain access to the services, but that the services provided are flexible enough to provide maximum continuity of care in the face of the transient life-style of some homeless people.

275 Purchasers will receive messages which do not always tally when they listen to the opinions of users as well as providers. This makes it all the more important that the strategy which guides purchasing is clear with regard to the kinds of services required, who they are for, and broadly, how they should operate. Strategies that make interchangeable reference to day centres, day hospitals or resource centres without any shared or more precise understanding of the purpose of these services, are more likely to run into the ground. Similarly, a commitment to purchase the services of particular workers will not by itself ensure an effective service. For example, in one area visited, the HAS found that the providers employed a commendably high number of community psychiatric nurses attached to GP surgeries. Nonetheless, the visiting team found little evidence that these CPNs had been encouraged to target their efforts on people in greater need, namely those with enduring serious mental illness, which includes some homeless people.

**276** In *Purchasing for Health*, it states that *"The purchaser-provider relationship cannot simply be restricted to formal negotiations.... it has to be constant and on-going. Both must realise that it is not a contest about who wins or loses in the negotiation process on contracts. A dialogue needs to be developed in which purchasers and providers jointly work to achieve their objectives."* This is pre-eminently so for the development of appropriate services for homeless mentally ill people.

**277** The organisational challenge facing purchasers can be summed up as falling into the following categories:

| | |
|---|---|
| **Strategic** | Deciding the level of need and how it will be delivered, and agreeing a multi-agency approach. |
| **Operational** | Measuring and monitoring need as a part of purchasing, contracting and training. |
| **Developmental** | Developments may be required in the internal organisation of purchasing organisations. The arrangements for organising strategic and operational change, defining responsibilities, and managing the process of change may all require adjustment to enable organisations to meet the needs of vulnerable groups in society. |

**278** Action at all levels of commissioning may be required if these organisational challenges are to be met. This will involve the authority members (values), executive directors (strategy) and operational managers (contracting, information and public health functions). Identification and implementation of a strategy for this client group may contribute to the agenda for, and process of, organisational development of commissioning and purchasing authorities.

# CHAPTER 12

*Developing Purchasing
Relationships*

## RESPONSIVENESS TO LOCAL PEOPLE

279    *"Discussions about the reforms are often dominated by issues of structure. It is all too easy to forget that the purpose of the reforms is not organisational perfection but to improve people's health. Patients and the public must have a say in health service decision-making."*

*Vision for Purchasing. Dr Brian Mawhinney.*

280    This section examines the issues of responsiveness and the importance of the voices of homeless people being heard in decision-making. All too often, people who are homeless are marginalised and disadvantaged. The voice of people who are homeless will not come across to health authorities without a commitment to listening, a commitment to providing relevant information to people who are homeless and a clear recognition that people who are homeless are part of the population and have a right of equity of access to all health services.

281    There are a number of key factors which make the involvement of homeless people, particularly those with mental health problems, a different and more difficult task.

- People who are homeless cannot be seen in a straightforward way as 'patients' because of their difficulties of gaining access to the system.

- Frequently, people who are homeless have had bad past experiences of the psychiatric system and are wary of statutory services.

- The health service is gradually developing a capacity to listen to the views of mental health service users. There has been rapid and promising development in recent years and the task is not an easy one if tokenism and superficial answers are to be avoided. Much remains to be achieved in many areas.

- The interests of people who are homeless and who have mental health problems are different to those of the general public. Their primary concerns are not long waiting lists or the failure of outpatient clinics to keep appointment times. Their overriding concerns are for shelter, food and money.

- Homeless people are harder to contact and to engage in carrying out opinion surveys. It is unlikely that they will attend public meetings, join local health forums or use telephone hotlines.

282    Despite the HAS experience of one or two areas that were visited in the course of the service visits, where there is a consistent effort from purchasers to involve users of mental health services at all levels of planning, there is little evidence of any specific attention being made to attempt to involve the homeless user population. In areas where there are specialist teams working with homeless people with mental health problems, the experience of users is that they are listened to and that services are responsive to their needs. However, the existence of specialist teams did not of itself appear to ensure that homeless people had any voice in purchasing decisions in the area.

283    The examples of best practice came from areas where there was more acknowledgement of the needs of homeless people and where link workers had been employed by the local authority or the health authority or the voluntary sector to work with homeless people. There are a variety of different models. In some areas, health visitors or community psychiatric

*"All they can do is tell you to pull yourself together when you are pulling your hair out and banging your head against a brick wall."*

*Quote from user*

nurses are employed to offer services directly to homeless people. In other areas, there are health care co-ordinators who approach users in a planned way to arrange service packages in response to identified need.

284    There were two areas that stood out in terms of their response to homeless people with mental health problems. One has a voluntary sector team which does commendable work in enabling homeless people to gain access to services. In the other, the example is of a team of clinical staff who work directly with homeless people with mental health problems. In both areas, a feature central to the role of these teams is that they work alongside the mainstream statutory services to establish improved responses to this client group.

*"There was complete disregard of two voluntary sector documents on housing and homelessness by decision-making bodies."*

*Quote from user visitor report*

285    The pattern of provision across the country is that it is generally, but not exclusively, the voluntary sector that is providing services which are accessible and appropriate to the homeless population. In many cases, these agencies try to improve access to the health service for homeless people. This is a function which agencies attempt to achieve at both organisational and individual service user levels. In this way, these agencies apply certain pressure to develop more responsive mainstream services. Some voluntary agencies are taking the initiative to encourage the development of GP surgeries in community projects in order to facilitate access. At an individual level they provide considerable informal advocacy work for homeless people who need services.

286    In the present circumstances, it seems likely that the traditional role of the voluntary sector as the major provider of services for homeless people is likely to continue. This has important implications for statutory services. They should be responsive to requirements asked of them by voluntary workers - for example, by making referrals, or when seeking an assessment of need - and they should recognise the levels of experience and skill which are often found among voluntary sector providers. During the service visits, HAS visiting teams were repeatedly told by voluntary workers about their feelings of frustration when trying to make contact with statutory services.

*"Everyone feels the same but they're frightened to complain in case they lose the little they've got."*

*Quote from user*

287    It is important for NHS staff to be aware that the health service is often seen as impenetrable by voluntary sector organisations. The purchaser-provider system is still seen as confusing and often agencies do not know where to take their concerns. Repeatedly, HAS teams were given the opinion that meetings and discussions never led to any action. In situations in which finance came from statutory sources, an additional concern was reported that this might compromise the advocacy role of the agency.

288    Conversely, HAS teams also heard frequent references to the value placed by purchasers upon the advocacy functions of the voluntary sector, and of their wish to incorporate these into the planning and operation of services. There were a number of examples of their co-ordinating voluntary sector agencies or of Community Health Councils establishing forums on homelessness, and others in which agencies were brought together to identify gaps in services. Nevertheless, the general view given was one of a poor response to the client group by the statutory sector.

289    Where consultation did take place with the voluntary sector, the HAS detected that there was a tendency for purchasers to talk to the biggest voluntary sector provider in the area and for this to be seen as completing

the task of discussion. But, as cited earlier, the homeless population is increasingly a very diverse one. It includes women, young people, elderly people, black and minority ethnic people and refugees and many of these small groups of homeless people may lack effective contacts with the larger organisations. Many agencies in the voluntary sector reported that they do not feel accessible to all of those groups and that they are often dominated by a traditional clientele of older white men. Other people who are homeless tend to use community groups, church groups, women's groups, young people's centres or they are out of touch with services altogether. It is important that the diversity of the homeless population and the broad nature of the voluntary sector is taken into account when purchasers look at local needs.

290 Keeping in touch with this sector, understanding the issues for their user population, improving their awareness of health issues, and keeping them informed about the health service, is not a job that can be done informally as part of the task of clinical workers. Networking with community groups, understanding their information and service needs, and giving them a voice in planning and purchasing, is a vital task and it should be built into the structure of health authority commissioning action plans. HAS visiting teams found commendable examples of the voluntary sector involvement at this level, but these seemed to be exceptional. However, consulting with, listening and responding to the concerns of the voluntary sector should not be taken as satisfying the need for consultation with homeless people.

291 The HAS Thematic Review *Suicide Prevention - The Challenge Confronted* provides information on a range of contract models appropriate to formalising relationships between the voluntary and statutory sectors.

## Consulting Service Users

292 For all the reasons given earlier, consulting with people who are homeless with mental health problems is difficult. This is a task that may have to be developed slowly and in stages. The first requirement is a commitment to respecting and taking seriously the views of homeless people who experience mental health problems and illness. There are various possible ways of approaching the task.

- Health authorities could work alongside voluntary sector agencies. Their contracts might agree that providers which work closely with the homeless population should run discussion groups on their behalf to find out about users' views.

- Health authorities might commission local research into the needs of their homeless population which includes identification of users' views in the research specification.

- Health authorities could provide resources for local mental health users' forums, and ask them to carry out work to discover the views of homeless users.

- Health authorities could ensure that patient satisfaction surveys take into account the fact that some people are homeless, and are sensitive to their interests. For instance, monitoring satisfaction with care programming and discharge arrangements should always take into account the possibility of patients not having their own homes. These patients should be asked about how well they felt account was

*"Many people didn't know what an advocate was, but, when it was explained to them, said they would like one."*

*Quote from user visitor report*

*"When you're ill, simple issues become major ones. Practical problems get no help."*

*"What we need is a real job."*

*Quotes from user*

taken of this matter. This example also indicates the importance of involving users in their own care planning.

- Health authorities should ensure that some provision is assigned to fast-track assessments.

293 It is important to recognise the linguistic and racial diversity of the homeless population. Refugees who have arrived recently in this country, often following trauma, bereavement and separation from their family and friends, are particularly likely to be homeless and may be experiencing mental health problems. In order to be responsive to the added disadvantages of language difficulties and racism which may be encountered by refugees and people from black and minority ethnic groups, health authorities should develop equal opportunities strategies which consider issues such as:

- the employment of staff which reflect the diverse cultural and ethnic make-up of the local area;

- ethnic monitoring;

- training for staff in order that they can recognise and cater for different cultural, religious and dietary requirements;

- availability of interpreters and translated information, including their availability in out-of-hours provision;

- availability of health advocates.

294 Anecdotally, it has been said that health is a lesser priority for people who are homeless. If this were true, it cannot be a reason for the health service to give lower priority to their needs. Rather, it should urge the health service to understand the true priorities of homeless people, and respond to their health needs in a way that takes these into account. Some of the key concerns of homeless people who experience mental health problems are the same as other users of mental health services, and the latter are now increasingly well documented. Other concerns are directly related to their homeless status, and their need for housing, food and money.

*"The feeling is that, if you are homeless, you should be grateful for what you are given and should not really expect a choice of services. . ."*

*Quote from user visitor report*

295 During the service visits, some users of services reported their clear feelings that, because they are homeless, they are expected to be grateful for anything they are given and that they should not expect a choice of services or for services to be offered in clean and decent environments. Where homeless people are offered well-planned and well-designed housing and support services they feel real improvements can be achieved in their state of mental health. Restoration of their dignity and stability in their lives enable some people to change to lower doses of medication and to think about exploring their potential for work and independent living. Conversely, the lack of appropriate housing is seen by a number of people as a major factor in their relapse.

296 Poverty is the common experience of many of the homeless users who were contacted. Simple measures, like the provision of a bus pass, help people who cannot afford bus fares. For some, this service has been a lifeline enabling them to get to day centres and drop-ins or to see friends. A more complex issue concerns the level of benefits people who live in registered care homes are awarded. In some instances this is a powerful disincentive to people in need of accommodation with support to their taking up the option of accommodation which, in other ways, would meet their needs.

297 Issues of housing and finance are not the remit of the health service. Nonetheless, provision of a health service, which is responsive and attractive to this client group, often requires the provision of advice on a range of parallel and non-health service issues. NHS purchasers and providers should take account of these priorities in designing services and in responding to their users.

298 Homeless people also require services that respond out-of-hours, ie at times when they are most likely to experience a crisis and need support. Additionally, homeless people need places to go to in the daytime which offer company and constructive activities, food, laundry and washing facilities. They require access to counselling services and to advocacy services. Some homeless people have reported an awareness that their own feelings of anger turning to aggression can make their access to services even more difficult, and that advocacy could help them to get the support and services they need.

### Key Issues In Ensuring Services are Responsive to the Local Population

Certain imperatives emerge for health service commissioners:

- Listen to voluntary sector agencies working with homeless people; respond to their needs as an agency and the needs of the individuals with whom they are working.

- Recognise the diversity of the homeless population and the agencies that they use.

- Develop equal opportunities strategies which recognise the particular needs of refugee and black and minority ethnic homeless people.

- Encourage the establishment of forums for agencies working with homeless people. Consider providing financial support for these forums and supporting them with information and time as they, in turn, are a useful resource for gaining information on the needs of the homeless population.

- Negotiate with providers and encourage them to employ clinical link workers to work directly with the homeless population or to employ advocates for homeless people to link them into services. The choice requires determination of a model which best fits the area.

- Build into local services a recognition that homeless people have priorities other than for health services. They may need time to be spent on working with them on benefits or housing issues.

### MATURE RELATIONSHIPS WITH PROVIDERS

299 The development of the purchaser-provider system has emphasised the distinction between the roles of health authorities and provider units. This requires health service providers to adapt to a new role in which they no longer take the lead in service strategy development, as this is a clear commissioning function, though they clearly retain a key responsibility for contributing to the work of commissioners in this respect.

300 In spite of this role differentiation in this new relationship, long-term partnerships, based on long-term agreements, must remain. The use of

*"There appeared to be a commitment to ensure that housing is important to community care planning. It was apparent that improved inter-agency communication and planning would benefit homeless people."*

*Quote from user visitor report*

*"So it was good to know that he could have at least one hot meal a day and see a member of the medical profession when needed. He could also obtain clothing and wash his clothes and change there. He also used the bathing facilities."*

*"We don't want to be told to 'sit down, shut up', we want a laugh and a joke."*

*"People like to have animals and babies around."*

*"We need to feel happy."*

*Quotes from user visitor report*

longer-term (rolling) contracts, particularly with voluntary agencies, is likely to enable good working relationships to develop. These may be slow to develop, as each organisation establishes itself in its new role and may be especially so if organisations with the independent sector, who do not usually work with health service commissioners, are involved.

301   If they are to have lasting value and credibility, the contracts should be agreed with the clinical staff in the provider organisations, who deliver services, as well as between managers in the two organisations. Experience shows that this goes a long way towards ensuring that the contracts are realistic and effective in delivering their stated objectives.

302   More direct links between clinical staff and public health staff, or other clinically trained staff in purchaser organisations, should be fostered. These may be aided by purchaser organisations directly employing staff who have clinical backgrounds to take the lead in developing new service contracts.

303   It is important that relationships between purchasers and providers are sustained through regular contact, so that issues which effect quality are considered through routine monitoring and services can be adjusted accordingly.

304   There are opportunities for joint agency developments over purchasing and providing services for homeless people, and investment should be made in joint training involving all the relevant agencies. The effectiveness of these relationships - involving workers, professionals and managers - is critical in delivering a high quality service. Effort should also be made to foster and develop good long-term relationships between providers in an emerging broader spectrum of providers. This includes recognition of the requirements for networking between staff in all the organisations through to its inclusion in service specifications. The time required for these relationships to develop should be recognised in contract prices.

## LOCAL ALLIANCES

305   Clinical treatment, social care and housing, provided singly, are not likely to give adequate cover for people whose needs are so complex and so strongly inter-related. Formal and informal alliances will better ensure the delivery of a service which reduces the risk of admission and re-admission to hospital, as well as complaints and protests by neighbours and the general public. This enables a seamless pattern of care, provided by the most appropriate people.

306   The multiple and complex needs of most homeless mentally ill people can challenge the capacity of all agencies. The active formation of local alliances helps to ensure that this group of people receives a comprehensive and appropriate service. Alliances at local level are needed at all stages: for information gathering and sharing; for strategic and operational planning; for the commissioning and provision of services; and for training.

307   These alliances should be based upon principles of mutual respect, trust and open-mindedness between agencies and individuals. This acknowledges the skills, experience, resources and responsibilities which each partner in the alliance brings to the task. The range of potential stakeholders in the provision of services for homeless people is very wide,

and the importance of developing and nurturing alliances should be recognised. Stakeholders include: GPs; housing departments; voluntary agencies (including housing associations); the police; probation services; and drug and alcohol misuse and advisory agencies. This is not an exhaustive list, and the range will vary between localities. It is important that the role and contribution of all potential and actual service providers, though many are not designated as providing mental health services, is not overlooked by purchasing authorities.

308    The potential partners in local alliances are listed in Table 9.

*Table 9*

| Potential Partners in Local Alliances |
| --- |
| • Agencies which provide services for people who misuse drugs, alcohol and other substances |
| • Social services departments |
| • District/borough housing departments |
| • Health authorities |
| • GP fundholders |
| • General practitioners (non-fund holding) and other members of primary health care teams |
| • Health service provider units |
| • Voluntary sector umbrella groups, eg the Councils of Voluntary Service |
| • Probation services |
| • The police |
| • Mental health voluntary agencies, eg MIND, the National Schizophrenia Fellowship |
| • Local colleges and universities |
| • User groups - local and national |
| • Housing associations |
| • Churches |
| • Community Health Councils |
| • Residents and tenants associations |
| • Local press, radio, and TV |
| • Private sector home owners |

309    Assessment of need under the care in the community legislation is an activity in which formal alliance building could be particularly fruitful. The HAS service visits identified some useful examples in which appropriate statutory or voluntary agencies were given delegated powers by local authority social services departments to carry out, on their behalf, individual assessments in settings used by homeless people. Carrying this one stage further, some voluntary agencies, working with drug and alcohol misusers, are being given the financial revenue, via joint commissioning and

contracting with the health and social services, to allow them to make direct purchases of appropriate care for their clients. This too appears to be working very satisfactorily and has the full support of the statutory authorities concerned. The HAS thematic review - *Suicide Prevention, the Challenge Confronted* - contains relevant material on mechanisms for contracting with the voluntary sector.

310 The service visits also indicated, repeatedly, how much of the information on homelessness in terms of type, incidence and location, lay within the voluntary sector agencies. Such information is not always available in quantifiable form, but the HAS teams' interviews with project workers, in all the areas visited, yielded a far fuller picture of people's needs, and especially of their problems in gaining access to mental health, drug and alcohol services. Teams were also told that voluntary bodies are seldom asked for information on these matters, at either planning stages or in the measurement of activity levels. In any meaningful survey of need, the importance at the strategic level of seeking and sharing information, both statistical and descriptive, cannot be overstated.

## Health and Housing

311 Health service commissioners can benefit from early discussions with the relevant departments on the strategic and operational plans of the local authorities. A key element of influence on this particular alliance is the quality of the relationship between social services and housing personnel. Some areas have established multi-disciplinary panels for the assessment of vulnerability under the Housing Act 1985. These panels operate in differing ways, but commonly they include representatives from housing and social services departments and sometimes a health service representative. They make decisions on vulnerability and try to arrange appropriate support for homeless people. Where these panels are in operation, effective joint working is reported and more appropriate placements of single homeless people with mental health problems result. Where social services and housing departments are working well together, health purchasers are more likely to be in the picture. Where, as in a few areas, housing and social services operate as a unitary department, this also fosters healthy co-working. Little evidence was found of district and borough housing departments having any input into long-term planning. Instead, the HAS teams found that all too often housing officers learn of the impending discharge from hospital of patients a few hours before it happens and they are, therefore, often unable to respond effectively.

## Special Posts to Nurture Alliances

312 Alliances do not develop spontaneously. The HAS visiting teams were impressed by the effect of the financial investment of the statutory services in specially created posts designed to develop and maintain networks in mental health care, including those in services for homeless people. These posts are found in both the statutory and voluntary sectors and they have been found to add value through the development of healthy working partnerships and an atmosphere of trust. The existence of these networking posts has maximised the effectiveness of the Mental Illness Specific Grant (MISG) in some of the areas visited by the HAS where its imaginative allocation has improved the access to services of homeless mentally ill people. This has been achieved by appointing link workers and community psychiatric nurses to work with them.

## Joint Training

313   Training is an essential tool in fostering a shared understanding of need and common values system. The importance of inter-agency training to the field of mental illness services for homeless people is strengthened if it is extended to, for example, the police and the probation service. Good work is done in a number of districts where the police, health providers and social services co-operate in the formulation of operational policies on the use of Section 136 of the Mental Health Act 1983 and the Police and Criminal Evidence Act (PACE) 1984; also on the use of accident and emergency units as places of safety. Joint training underpins developments of this kind and paves the way for the more challenging development of court diversion schemes for mentally disordered offenders, many of whom have no permanent address. The integration of staff, who work with homeless people in an outreach capacity, with the staff of these diversion schemes is proving very effective in at least one London area.

## Involving the Private Sector

314   The private sector is often a provider of services, but is seldom regarded as an active partner in a similar way as voluntary agencies. Where extensive use is made of bed and breakfast establishments by hospital and social services staff, concern is often expressed about the quality of care offered to vulnerable residents. Landlords and landladies can become valued partners in provision if they are offered training and continuing support in their role as carers. The introduction of some kind of system of accreditation for bed and breakfast homes (where the Residential Homes Act 1984 may not apply) is one way of encouraging a partnership approach to care and of improving the quality of life of residents. This is an approach recommended by the HAS.

## Avoiding Fragmentation of Services

315   Internally, there is often an unnecessary separation or lack of contact between mental health, drug misuse and alcohol misuse services. There may be a lack of parity between these last two in terms of resources and priorities, and where this is the case, the possibility of a good working partnership is impeded. For homeless people with mental health problems, there is often a linked incidence of substance misuse and this emphasises the vital importance of effective liaison between different service elements. Similar observations may be made about the need for close collaboration between physical health care and mental health services.

## Working with Voluntary Organisations

316   The importance of the voluntary sector as a provider of services to homeless people has already been stressed in this report. The recent changes in the structure of both health and social services have increased this importance, and the need for creative working partnerships between statutory and non-statutory agencies is generally accepted as a positive and necessary approach.

317   In practice, however, the relationships between the two sectors are often less than creative. The HAS teams found that misconceptions of the other were held commonly by both types of agency. While there are a number of inaccurate stereotypes, there are true differences in culture, ethos and language between the statutory and voluntary sectors. These differences are upheld when there is little contact. Each side has much to contribute, however, and the more contact that is established, the more likelihood there is of challenging unhelpful preconceptions.

*"The mental health professionals don't see the voluntary sector as being professionals. They don't refer to the voluntary sector."*

*Quote from user visitor report*

318 Building and sustaining successful partnerships with voluntary organisations require considerable groundwork and mutual good will. The groundwork involves gaining knowledge about the ways in which the respective organisations and their staff work. In some cases, the professional training of people in the voluntary sector may be identical to that of their statutory colleagues. In others, there may be a differing range of long and valuable experience of working with particular groups of people. As has already been noted, voluntary agencies often operate within effective networks, giving them access to information, contacts and resources which are not necessarily directly available to the statutory sector. These assets can enable flexible and speedy responses to clients' needs.

*"There is not, however, a balanced pattern of long-term funding that gives voluntary agencies the security they need."*

*Quote from user visitor report*

319 Within the voluntary sector there are huge variations in capacity, size, skills and ways of working. With the advent of care in the community and changes in the health service, the larger voluntary agencies have begun to develop the skills necessary for them to enter into contractual partnerships. They have accepted the need for business plans, monitoring, evaluation, competent budgeting and accountability. In short, they are equipping themselves as valid providers of services, and many have adopted the language of the statutory sector. Smaller, more informal organisations may view these changes with concern, fearing that their aims and objectives could be compromised. So, it is reasonable, as part of the groundwork for developing partnerships, for the statutory authorities to devote time and interest to the voluntary agencies in order to enable them to acquire new management and contracting skills.

*"The bottom line is always money. Most existing funding is secured by established interests which are not delivering. Young organisations can collapse because of lack of administrative support, buildings and secure fundings."*

*Quote from user visitor report*

320 In brief, this bilateral process of laying the groundwork for enhanced relationships is summarised by Tables 10 and 11.

*Table 10*

| What Statutory Purchasers and Providers Need to Know About Voluntary Organisations |
| --- |
| • Which client groups do they serve? |
| • Who runs them? |
| • What is their management structure? |
| • What are their aims and objectives? |
| • Who funds them? |
| • What services do they provide? |
| • What is their catchment area? |
| • Are they financially viable? |
| • How accessible are they to clients? |
| • Do they operate within an equal opportunities framework? |
| • What are the skills and qualifications of staff? |
| • Are they familiar with contracting processes? |
| • Do the voluntary organisations have the capacity to expand? |
| • Do they attempt to involve service users in running their organisations? |

*Table 11*

| What Voluntary Organisations Need To Know As They Enter Into Partnerships With The Statutory Sector. |
|---|
| • Who are the key people in the statutory purchasing and providing agencies? |
| • What are their areas of responsibility? |
| • What are the commissioning and purchasing cycles? |
| • What arrangements are there for joint commissioning between the health and social services? |
| • What kind of contracts are being negotiated (eg, spot contracts, rolling contracts, yearly grants)? |
| • What kind of monitoring processes are required? |
| • Will core costs be recognised in contracts? |
| • Will training be available? |
| • Will any advocacy activities be in jeopardy? |

321 Where there is a co-ordinating agency such as a Council for Voluntary Service in an area, this is often a valuable starting point for statutory agencies wishing to develop operational links with the voluntary sector.

322 Partnerships with the voluntary sector often prosper when resources are pooled. The practices of GPs holding surgeries in drop-in centres, and of providing sessions by community psychiatric nurses or other clinicians in the premises of voluntary projects, may offer the best of both to the client. Providing other forms of health care, such as chiropody and dentistry, in the same setting can ensure that optimum use is made of a range of services.

323 Many voluntary organisations work with particular groups of people, and acquire much specialist knowledge in the process. This is especially the case in respect of agencies that work with black and different ethnic communities, including people who are refugees. Their expertise is very valuable both to users, providers of direct services, and, as a resource, to mainstream statutory agencies. Such organisations may, however, be quite small in scale and unversed in the intricacies of negotiation and contracting. So, reciprocally, link workers from the statutory sector, for example psychiatric nurses or health visitors, can help to establish good working links and develop mutual trust in parallel with providing services to users.

324 Voluntary agencies may be involved in work at a variety of levels and stages, eg their early involvement in strategic planning, collaboration on the more detailed work of developing individual projects, and co-working in established focused schemes. All of these can enrich the quality of service delivery. This may be particularly important for homeless people who may be in touch with community groups, but have little contact with the mainstream statutory services.

*"The social and psychological problems faced by some users are serious but, with the right resources and help, certainly not insurmountable."*

*Quote from user visitor report*

*"Social workers never come near us. I think they're frightened of the users."*

*Quote from hostel worker*

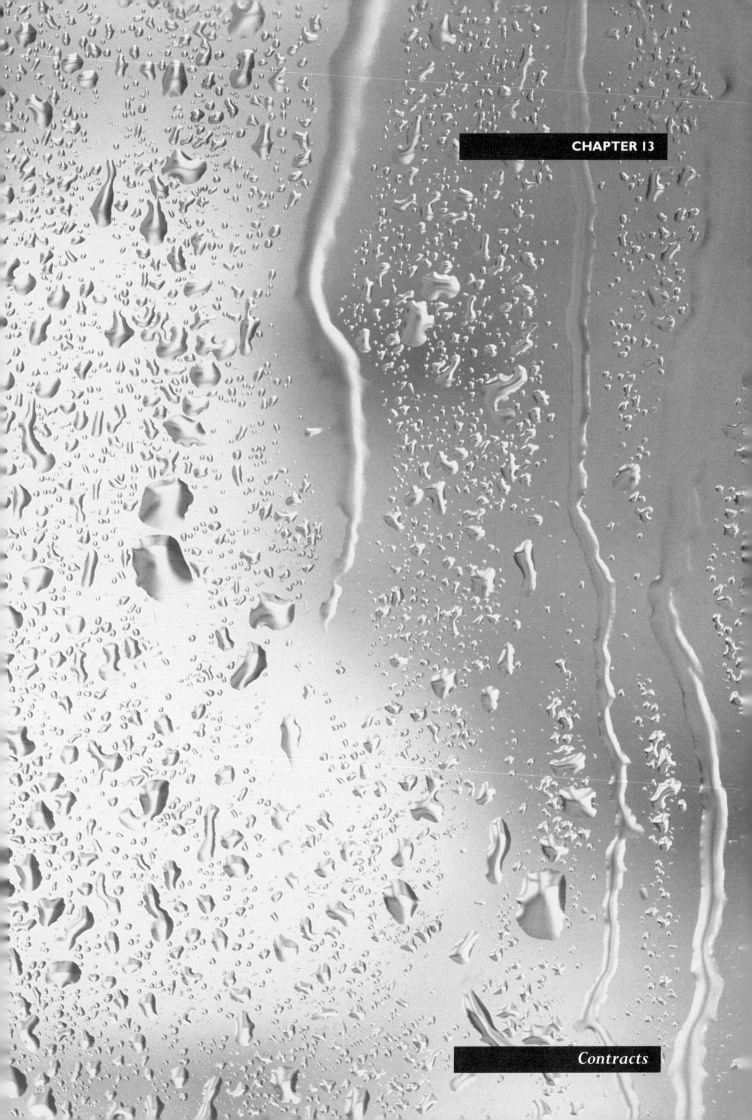

**CHAPTER 13**

*Contracts*

## EFFECTIVE CONTRACTS FOR SERVICES FOR MENTALLY ILL PEOPLE

325    Seven imperatives for effective contracting were identified in *Purchasing for Health*. These are:

- Better working between purchasers and providers

- Involvement of doctors in the contracting process

- Involvement of nurses in the contracting process

- Realism about activity and the impact of change

- Ensuring contracts are appropriate

- Effective monitoring arrangements

- Robust information on activity and prices

They apply to all health services and, thus, equally to mental health services for homeless people.

326    Throughout this report, the authors use the term 'clinical staff' to include all relevant professionals. Thus, the second and third items in the list above have been expanded to reflect an appropriate approach to the subject.

### Better Working between Purchasers and Providers

327    A key issue for homeless mentally ill people is that of achieving a unity of purpose across the range of different purchasers in an area. This includes NHS purchasers (health authorities and family health services authorities [until 1996], and GP fundholders), social services departments, and housing departments. Good communication between all purchasers and providers across the sectors is an important corollary of this principle. Evidence was gained in the HAS service visits of hierarchical management structures in some provider agencies that inhibited the flow of communication between managers and staff and which acted as a barrier to effective response to the needs of homeless people with mental health problems. This was particularly important where specific service provision for this client group was fragmentary or absent. In negotiating contracts for access to mainstream services, homeless people generally, and mentally ill homeless people specifically, are frequently overlooked in the existing contractual arrangements between purchasers and providers. Seven out of 10 of the purchasers visited in the fieldwork had not included any reference to homeless people in their contract specifications and the same number was unable to determine if there were any problems with service uptake for this group since it was not monitored.

328    Better working in this context will require health authorities to enter into arrangements for services for the client group with private and voluntary sector providers or to agree joint arrangements with other purchasers such as social services and housing departments or FHSAs. Where the voluntary sector is already working in an organised way with mentally ill homeless people, it is frequently more efficient to link into those services that are already provided. Purchasers should ensure that they have good information about the roles, quality of work and experience of voluntary sector agencies so that they can make informed decisions when considering tenders for contracts.

329  When working with non-NHS providers, purchasers and sub-contracting providers may need to recognise that small or newly established voluntary organisations may require help to set up and manage the contracting process. Investment of time, spent in preliminary discussion with staff and managers in the voluntary sector, is likely to enhance working relationships and promote variety in service provision.

330  A long lead time to achieve effective service delivery is not unusual when working with some mentally ill homeless people, particularly those who may have been street homeless or long-term hostel dwellers. Purchasers should recognise that clinicians who work with homeless people should carry smaller case loads. Nonetheless, rapid crisis intervention may be required for other clients, so contracts and the range of services offered should be sufficiently flexible to enable the issues arising from the fluctuations in the size and characteristics of the client group to be managed.

331  Networking of services is essential and involves work across local NHS and social services, as well as across other geographical, boundaries. The service visits conducted by the HAS revealed impressive examples of services which have been established and are thriving in such networks. Equally, examples were found where, for the want of such sensitive working, homeless individuals were failing to receive necessary services.

332  On a number of occasions, fieldwork teams were told by voluntary sector providers that they felt that they made all the running, and that relationships with health service providers were one-sided rather than reciprocal. Where positive relationships were found, this was generally because purchasers had devoted time to visiting projects for homeless people, familiarising themselves with the work, as well as discussing both quality and contractual issues.

333  These informal initiatives can be reinforced by more formal structures. In several of the service visits, specially designated posts for liaison workers were found within the statutory sector. These postholders were evidently proving to be effective co-ordinators in brokering relationships between statutory sector purchasers and non-statutory providers.

334  The development of such structures depends on building long-term relationships between service providers and purchasers and, when voluntary sector partners are involved, on ensuring a degree of stability in the financing arrangements for those partners. Rolling contracts, eg over three years, are more likely to achieve stability of this kind.

**Involving Clinical Staff in the Contracting Process**

335  All relevant clinical staff should be involved in the contracting process for this client group, in addition to doctors and nurses. Thus, psychologists, occupational therapists, health visitors, chiropodists and dentists should contribute their experience and expertise. The HAS service visits indicated that, in a number of areas, it is the consultant psychiatrists who are the clinicians most evidently missing from the contracting process. Commissioners should ensure that they are invited to discussions alongside provider managers.

**336** To enable satisfactory and effective contracts to be set for the client group, it is essential to involve those clinical staff who deliver services in the agreement of the objectives for the service and the targets for monitoring it so that contracts are tangible and set to achieve real and appropriate goals rather than all-embracing objectives. The service visits provided evidence of areas where purchasers had developed their contracts without the involvement of any other agency. There were also places where the voluntary sector and users had been consulted but where the provider staff who were asked to meet the targets set had not been consulted, and did not know that the contracts existed.

**337** It is clear from the experience of the HAS that the most effective contracts are those which are owned by all three parties – purchasers, providers and representatives of users – and where there is a joint commitment to seeing them achieve their aims.

**338** A key element for purchasers is ensuring that GP fundholders and non-fundholders are fully involved so that access to primary and secondary care is maintained. Development of service specifications is a critical element that requires the active involvement of purchaser and provider clinicians if contracts are to be realistic.

**Realism about Activity and the Impact of Change**

**339** Service delivery for homeless people provides a particular challenge for measurement of activity. The experience of the HAS indicates that a starting point might be that of agreeing a methodology for measuring the housing status of persons seen in community mental health services, in accident and emergency departments, drug and alcohol treatment units and for inpatients admitted to mental health services, in order to assess the nature of use made of existing services. Such a system for monitoring housing status must be more sophisticated than the current monitoring of people who are of no fixed abode.

**340** A model that has been recommended is to ask all patients where they live and then to give them a list of accommodation types from which to choose. This might include:

- Owned/rented flat/house

- Staying with friends, relatives or parents, by choice

- Staying with friends, relatives or parents against own wishes

- Local authority temporary accommodation

- Bed and breakfast hotel (DSS funded)

- Bed and breakfast hotel (as a tourist)

- Hostel

- Squat

- Night shelter

- Sleeping out

- Traveller

- Other (please specify)

This list is an example; some categories may not be relevant in some localities while others may need to be added to reflect local conditions.

341    The use made of services by people who are in the differing categories of homelessness should be compared with the local levels of homelessness, calculated from the indicators discussed earlier in this chapter and with the projected level of referral to specialist services from such a population.

*"It was felt that if homeless people tried to access services, their immediate needs would not be met. All felt their contact with homeless people was inadequate and would require some effort, even to provide a minimal service."*

*Quote from user visitor*

342    Generally, improving access to mental health care will involve training staff in the providing agencies which, in turn, should promote positive shifts in the attitudes of staff towards homeless mentally ill people.

343    It is vital that change is planned in consultation with providers. Staff who monitor housing status should be given an explanation of the reasons for this task and training and support should be made available. Time should be taken to achieve the co-operation of staff. Better systems of recording housing status will change perceptions and thereby increase the number of homeless people seen. It is likely that these changes will be followed later by changes in activity levels.

344    Some service outputs are difficult to measure in respect of this client group. For example, when conducting outreach work with street homeless people, the number of contacts will not directly indicate the nature or quality of service offered. Some clients may require intensive work on an outreach basis before formal entry to treatment may occur. This can take weeks or months rather than days.

345    In the HAS service visits, some authorities expressed anxiety about delivery of services creating its own demand. This kind of magnet effect did not seem to be substantiated in practice. In the populations of all the authorities visited, it was possible to identify groups of homeless people with mental health problems. It also became clear that, where there are well planned and accessible services for homeless mentally ill people, there is likely to be a decreased demand for acute services which require more intensive and higher cost interventions.

**Ensuring Contracts are Appropriate**

346    Contracts should be appropriate to the services which are purchased and they must also be consistent with the providers' capacity to generate and record meaningful information. It is particularly important that contracts for services for mentally ill homeless people, whether these are part of generic mental health services or partly provided by specialist services geared to mentally ill homeless people specifically, should be centred on the patient/ user.

347    In *Purchasing for Poverty*, Access to Health produced a guide to commissioning health services for homeless people which sets out six areas for which targets and statements should be developed in all contracts. The areas are:

**Access**          - Equity
                    - Staff attitudes
                    - Advocacy/interpreting
                    - Transport

| | |
|---|---|
| **Flexibility** | - Self-referral |
| | - Appointment times |
| | - Outreach work |
| | - Hand-held records |
| | - Multi-disciplinary approach |
| **Training** | - For health staff |
| | - For the staff of agencies that offer services to homeless people |
| **Information** | - Provided at places to which homeless people go |
| | - For staff about local services for homeless people |
| **Monitoring and Evaluation** | - Use of services by homeless people |
| | - Outcomes for homeless users of services |
| **Multi-agency work** | - Ensuring co-ordinated provision of services across agencies |

**348** Evidence from the service visits conducted by the HAS also showed the importance of networking with other agencies that work with homeless people in the same area. The HAS has come to the opinion that this should be a specific responsibility which should also appear in service specifications.

**349** Contracts which are sensitive to the needs of homeless people for services can be achieved either by a separate specification, appended to all relevant contracts, or by referring to the needs of homeless people within each appropriate contract. The document *Purchasing and Poverty* provides greater detail and gives examples of the targets that can be developed.

**350** Acceptability of services to users is a key target. The views of users on the services in the authorities visited indicate that, in a number of authorities, homeless people found significant problems in obtaining access to mental health services and also to drug and alcohol detoxification facilities. Users emphasised the need for advocacy services for homeless people with mental health problems.

**351** Properly addressed, contracts for this client group can help to meet the Health of the Nation targets for reduction in the level of suicide, since homeless people have higher rates of suicide than the general population.

### Robust information on Activity and Prices

**352** Local variations and historical factors make it difficult to establish useful indicators for monitoring service contracts for homeless mentally ill people. Such variations also make it more demanding to determine service costs.

**353** To tackle circumstances of this kind, purchasers need to agree levels of local service activity with providers, as well as appropriate contract prices. Given the marginalisation of the client group, it may be worthwhile for purchasers to separate or earmark particular expenditure for homeless people within their service contracts. Service targets should be shared, explicit and realistic.

## MONITORING AND CONTRACT LEVERS

**354** All these factors underline how important it is for commissioners to establish a strategic approach to homeless mentally ill people. Integral to this strategic approach, purchasers must develop an understanding of local issues, purchase accordingly and establish appropriate and realistic monitoring. Obviously, contracting alone cannot develop services. Among other things, the contracting process should be used to confirm the agreement and implementation of strategic objectives.

**355** It is also important for commissioners to establish the context in which they purchase. Areas to assess include: the purchasers' role; their relationships with providers (in both the statutory and voluntary sectors); purchasing approach; and other priorities.

**356** Targets in service specifications should be linked to performance indicators that are easily measurable, unambiguous and relevant to homeless mentally ill people.

**357** A checklist of specific requirements relating to homeless people might include:

- Definition of the target groups within the client population, eg street homeless people and/or those in short-term accommodation such as direct access hostels.

- Liaison with other agencies - especially primary care, mental health services, alcohol and drug misuse services.

- Written agreements and protocols for access to psychiatric and medical advice and care.

- Agreed statements concerning the relationships between accident and emergency services and other services, with respect to homeless mentally ill people, and statements concerning the role of accident and emergency services with people who are homeless, whether or not mentally ill.

- Statements concerning the agreed levels of direct work with people who have alcohol and drug-related health problems or illnesses.

- An agreement to undertake assessments and to provide care in line with the requirements of the Mental Health Act 1983.

- Estimates of the requirements placed on providers for their staff to be involved in the arrangements concerning the housing and/or resettlement of homeless people.

- An agreement for statutory sector providers to offer training to voluntary sector staff on care planning, health and housing issues.

**358** Monitoring should be carried out by both purchaser and provider. An alternative is for purchasers to use the services of a third party to monitor some areas of service delivery. This approach is a valuable spur to the development of advocacy services for this client group. However, the experience of the HAS is that good quality monitoring is usually best led by providers. Generally, the HAS recommends that commissioners should avoid setting standards, wherever possible, but should require providers to set their own standards and performance indicators and then provide proper monitoring information. Propelled in this way, monitoring can gain the whole-hearted involvement and support of provider staff.

359  In certain circumstances, contracts may need to specify incentives and penalties relating to contract performance. Incentives may take a number of forms. For example, continuation of a rolling contract could depend on contract performance improving the long-term stability of the provider unit. Incentives could also be based on compliance with performance targets as agreed in service specifications.

## Steps to Effective Contracting

### Contract Setting

360  Two matters are of central significance:

- Ensuring that cost, volume and quality outcomes are clearly communicated.

- Developing monitoring and quality indicators that are meaningful.

### A Possible Checklist of Quality Indicators

361  The quality indicators suggested below reflect both the intention to promote readier access to services, and the views of users on the need for an holistic approach to their problems.

- The ability of the provider to meet the requirements of The Patients' Charter.

- The effective operation of an appropriate referral system. (Referral systems may be written or verbal and should be collaborative, involving the referrer, the service and the client.)

- The ability of specialist providers to complete a preliminary assessment within 48 hours of referral of all referred persons who are stated by their referrers to require this degree of urgent consideration.

- The allocation of a keyworker to clients where there is a need for longer-term support.

- Regular (eg three-monthly) reviews of every patient.

- Evidence of an holistic approach to assessment and care.

- The operation of effective equal opportunities policies, including the provision of services that are non-discriminatory, and those that are sensitive to the needs of women, people from black and ethnic communities, disabled people, gay men and lesbians.

- Evidence of the operation of a system for consulting service users on their own care, and on service developments.

### Performance Issues

362  Non-compliance or failure to meet identified goals may be due to a number of factors. Regular review of performance and audit of work will ensure that both purchasers and providers are aware of any changes or difficulties which have developed. In a situation where there is more than one potential provider, there may be some prospect of awarding contracts to other agencies, but this should be viewed as a last resort.

**Working with Providers**

363   A key factor for success is that of fostering long-term relationships between purchasers and providers. Short-term opportunistic purchasing is unlikely to provide effective and sensitive services for homeless people. A developmental approach is preferable, which ensures redefinition and reshaping of services, as required.

**Important Contracting Issues**

364   The following items summarise issues of central significance from this report.

- Targeted specialist approaches are effective in the short-term.

- GPs and secondary care specialist staff should be involved in developing the overall strategy.

- Clinicians within both secondary and primary care should be engaged in advising on contract objectives and targets, audit, training and research.

- Locally generated information is likely to provide valuable insights, and specific incentives directed at practice level are also important.

- It is important to share the development of strategy, which is then linked to shared working, and, if possible, to joint funding and commissioning with other agencies (eg social services and housing departments).

- There is considerable expertise in the non-statutory sector. A mixed pattern of provision based on expertise and effectiveness is more successful than limiting purchasing to agreements with single agencies.

365   Structure should always follow need, and form should follow function. Therefore, local patterns of provision, and by inference purchasing, may well vary considerably.

## A SUMMARY OF ADVICE TO COMMISSIONERS

366   The following are the core recommendations to commissioners:

- Establish a strategy that is shared with GPs and which has a local focus.

- Share the strategy and encourage working with other agencies, especially local authority departments.

- Ensure contracts are negotiated which confirm and implement the strategy, and that the strategy is not led by contracting.

- Develop a clear view of the local context for commissioning and purchasing.

- Adopt a collaborative approach to contracting with providers, using explicit targets and risk-sharing.

- Encourage positive approaches to contracting involving a mixed economy of providers from a range of sectors.

- Draw upon the views of users and voluntary agencies.

- Collaborate with clinicians on effective approaches.

- Consider positive incentives related to targeted work.

- Above all, ensure that commissioning is based on a health needs approach rather than a service-led approach.

- Meet providers' expectations of purchasers by:

    - developing a strategy which addresses better health, better health services and effective use of resources;

    - ensuring financial stability of services;

    - facilitating risk-sharing;

    - having an explicit short-term agenda, which is, preferably, shared;

    - being willing to innovate and underwrite programmes of change;

    - delivering what you say;

    - being prepared to exchange information freely as between service providers for contracts;

    - recognising that contracting is only part of the role;

    - being sensitive in planning change and securing it;

    - encouraging an approach to action planning that is based on continuous improvement;

    - balancing recurring and non-recurring investments;

    - encouraging excellence;

    - realising that each relationship is different;

    - expecting and anticipating changes in technical practice;

    - expecting resources to be maximised - focus on the difference between delivery and maximising potential;

    - encouraging providers to use their freedom.

## THE PRINCIPLES FOR MEASURING SUCCESS

367   Health service purchasers buy services to improve the health of their population; they should therefore purchase to improve the health care of homeless people in their districts. They should target resources to achieve the most effective ways of delivering care, based upon their existing knowledge.

368   The services they purchase for homeless people should be shown to improve the quality of their health care, and make it responsive and accessible to as many users as possible, and delivered in ways that users wish.

369   Purchasers should know that this is happening, not just by measuring inputs, such as budget size or numbers of staff employed, but also by systematic feedback from user surveys, involving the voluntary sector and using the knowledge of others.

370   A planned service will begin to achieve success if it considers working in all the following areas as part of an integrated approach to the needs of homeless people:

### Promotion

Are the services to homeless people promoted in the most appropriate ways? Is information available to all the agencies involved: hospitals; accident and emergency departments; GPs; and especially shelters, street agencies, and places where homeless people meet?

### Early Treatment

Many health problems affecting homeless people are chronic, under-detected and under-treated. Services should be available to allow screening and early treatment, and include full access to primary and secondary health care as soon as requested.

### Prevention

Active measures must be taken, including the provision of advice relating to drugs and alcohol, sexual health, general health, including self-care and diet, and advice on child care for single parents in temporary accommodation.

### Rehabilitation

Facilities should be available to allow homeless people to regain lost skills and restore stability and security. Stability of accommodation is needed before further rehabilitation can progress. Access to all mainstream rehabilitation services for mental illness, drug and alcohol-related disorders and to physical rehabilitation should be available and publicised.

## The Seven Guiding Principles

371  There are seven guiding principles for achieving success in purchasing health care (*Purchasing for Health*, 1993), and a service that is delivered well to a difficult and diverse group, such as homeless people, is more likely to deliver well to all other parts of its population. The principles are:

### Listen to the Service Users

How do they feel about the services, including their accessibility and availability, and staff attitudes? Are they aware of the services that are available? Standards such as those of The Patients' Charter apply to all the population including homeless people, so how do services for them measure up to the charter? Are the results of these comparisons available and published?

### Know What You Wish to Achieve

Clear targets are now defined in the Health of the Nation, and the objectives are applicable to homeless people. Local health authorities may also set their own local targets and priorities for homeless people. These targets should be based on good local information.

### Relate Service Contracts to Targets

Targets should be set in contracts for homeless people and should include those for the development and education of staff, the provision of information and health promotion as well as those for the delivery of assessment and treatment services.

*"It took them five months to recognise clinical depression and by then my marriage had gone out of the window."*

*"I had to wait two days for an appointment when I said I was suicidal."*

*"Who can I go to that will help? I was just floating on air. I told them I was suicidal and felt I was going to kill my child. It was a week before anyone visited."*

*Quotes from users*

*"It's no good putting people straight into long-term accommodation. They will only blow it. They need help in general living skills first in a supervised move-on place.*

*"Having a house doesn't solve everything. In some ways it's just a start."*

*Quote from user*

### Use Information on Effectiveness and Outcomes

A sound knowledge-base, including information, research and experience from elsewhere, will give purchasers the best chance to select the most effective clinical interventions, and the best preventive measures and models of service delivery applicable to homeless people.

### Use Contracts to Engage Providers in Health Promotion

Health care providers have a key role in health promotion, and for using their contacts with patients for screening, data collection and monitoring. By using their skills, expertise, existing good relationships and trust between staff in the field and homeless service users, opportunities for education and health promotion can be exploited.

### Use Local Clinical Audit Findings

Multi-disciplinary audit should take place in all organisations that provide services for homeless people. Audits of service use, outcomes, the implementation of the Care Programme Approach and service take-up by homeless people should be encouraged in the pursuit of improved services.

### Establish Challenging Efficiency Targets

Services should use scarce resources in the most efficient way, especially in areas of unmet need such as those for homeless people. Efficiency targets should be incorporated into the objectives for services.

The Implications for
Providers

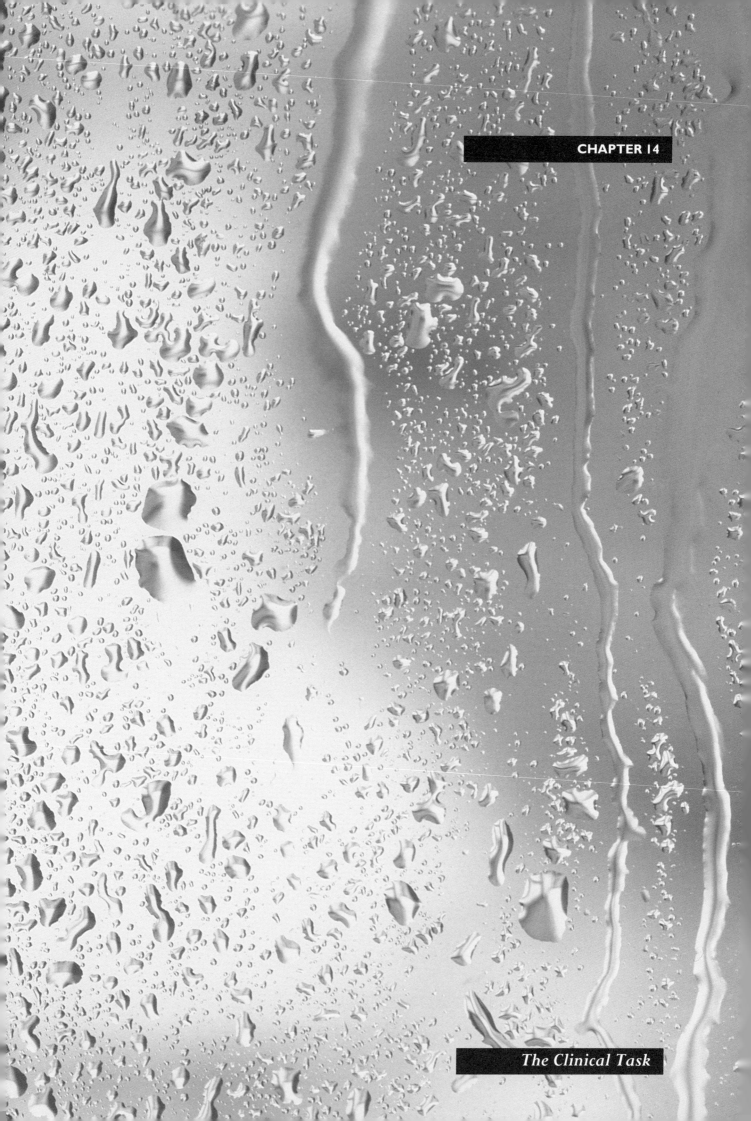

CHAPTER 14

*The Clinical Task*

## INTRODUCTION

372  It is more likely that a good quality mental health service that offers primary and secondary levels of care and is appropriate to the needs of people who are homeless will be provided by a service that is of high quality generally. Such a service will be fully comprehensive and responsive to the needs of its population. It must be able to demonstrate that it has strong working links with other agencies in the locality in the statutory and voluntary sectors.

373  It is unlikely that homeless people need access to long-term hospital care, but many have complex needs and well co-ordinated access to a broad-based community care system is important. Comprehensive community care involves both primary care practitioners and specialists working in a co-ordinated way alongside each other.

374  Some secondary level services offer a specialised team approach to this client group and others use existing mainstream services. Both approaches may be appropriate, if delivered and targeted effectively. Whichever style is preferred, it is likely that a specific clinical input is required, with more open access and ease of availability, to identify clients/patients and to refer them to the main body of a mainstream service.

## THE PRIMARY HEALTH CARE TASK

375  The primary health care system should be in a position to offer its services to homeless people. However, their access to primary care services is a problem because of their mobility and because homeless people present wide-ranging and often complex needs.

376  A variety of approaches to resolving this challenge has been tried, including dedicating GP sessions to homeless people, either on a paid sessional basis, or by practices being willing to set aside some of their clinic time for people who are not registered, to attend on an emergency basis. The disadvantage of the second approach is that it may only provide single consultations about particular problems, and not achieve continuity of care. The advent of GP fundholding is a challenge. It puts GPs in the position to achieve major improvements in services for homeless people.

377  Health authorities could place the responsibility for the provision of services for homeless people in fundholders' contracts. A more radical solution would be that of total fundholders using their purchasing power to purchase wide-ranging services, including social services and secondary care specialist services, for homeless people.

378  GPs should be involved in monitoring local care programme provision, and will then be able to influence the direction of services in response to local need. The key tasks for primary health care services is for their focused involvement with meeting the needs of homeless people.

379  Homeless people with mental health problems and disorders should make their presence felt most in the primary care setting. Most minor problems are managed without the need for referral to secondary mental health service providers. However, specialist mental health professionals - such as practice-based community psychiatric nurses, psychologists and counsellors - who work in primary health care settings need professional support to care adequately for homeless people.

380 Secondary mental health care providers need to know what services are available from local GP practices so that referral of, and responses to, the challenges of caring for homeless people can move in both directions. Close professional collaboration between primary and secondary service providers is especially important when working with homeless people.

## AWARENESS

381 Clinical staff who work in adult mental health services should have a competent level of awareness of the health issues associated with being homeless. This includes agreed operational definitions of the problem. These may be based on local definitions or those provided by statute.

382 Clinical staff should ensure that they use their local information systems both for updating their own activity appropriately and for planning and targeting their service activity. The information gathered should include the housing status of all clients within the system. Outreach services to shelters and to known street locations are important, as are those to areas of hidden homelessness, such as the residents of bed and breakfast accommodation, and those using day services provided for homeless mentally ill people. Target groups should include families with young children.

383 More specific aspects of awareness for service providers include the following:

- Staff in front-line areas, such as wards, clinics and resource centres, should be aware of the health needs of homeless people and should ensure their patients have access to the services they require. This should include access to primary health care services.

- The services offered should be non-stigmatising, and afford users some choice about where they are seen, if possible. Services delivered in a primary health care setting may be more acceptable to patients. Some services may need to be available in shelters and day units, given the reluctance of some users to use mainstream mental health services.

- There must be an acceptance that the health needs of homeless people may be complex, and involve physical as well as mental health issues.

- It is likely that traditional lines of referral, via primary health care practitioners, may not be appropriate or used, as many patients will not be registered with GPs. Clients may be more likely to gain access to services by other routes such as hospital accident and emergency departments, the police or self-presentation to components of specialist mental health services. Providers should be careful to avoid putting up unwitting barriers to their services. Frequently, these can include the routine conduct of out-of-hours assessment by junior medical staff. This reduces the chance of a full consultant or multi-disciplinary assessment for people who are referred by non-standard routes.

- Awareness may be increased if one consultant, or a clinical team in each mental health service, takes on responsibility for co-ordinating the mental health services for homeless people. This can offer clients a fast-track into the service rather than relying on traditional duty systems which may offer little clinical continuity to clients who repeatedly use the service.

- Liaison between health service staff, and with other agencies and workers in the field, is often easier when conducted or co-ordinated by one clinical team, although this must be balanced against the risk of ghettoising the problem.

- The staff who work in this specialised area should have access to a wide range of clinical skills, ranging from those appropriate to drug and alcohol problems to those required for responding to the complex needs of adult survivors of sexual abuse. It is important to remember that there is an increasing number of younger homeless people who may require specialised adolescent services.

- Staff, such as community psychiatric nurses, who work alone in the field and who may be employed by a range of agencies require regular access to clinical supervision and support. Even if not employed directly by the main health provider organisation, they should have access to one of the mental health teams, perhaps as honorary members, for peer support, ongoing education and professional development.

- Service delivery to homeless people should be considered as part of a regular clinical audit cycle. This might review the housing status of patients admitted to hospital (also emergency cases), the functioning of procedures established in respect of Section 117 of the Mental Health Act 1983, use of the Care Programme Approach, and the use made by homeless people of regular clinics and mental health resource centres. Ideally, audits of these kinds should be linked with other quality measures, such as user surveys.

## RELATIONSHIPS

384   Homeless people go for help to many agencies because of their multiple needs, and the voluntary sector is often the main provider or co-ordinator of services and support. The development of close working relationships between the health, housing and social services, the police and probation services and the voluntary sector, is therefore essential.

385   There are certain specific issues that concern relationships:

- The traditional relationship, in which the voluntary sector is seen as the junior partner with the health service, may need to be reversed. Sometimes, health service workers may need to acknowledge the superior experience of voluntary sector workers in this field, and their wider knowledge of the problems and appropriate solutions.

- Specialist workers, such as community psychiatric nurses, who work with homeless people, should have close working relationships with inpatient wards and community services, in order to ensure that their patients are able to gain easy access to the services they need. Many of their clients will have no GP, so access to specialist services via this route may not be possible. Services should not turn clients away because they are not referred by a GP. It may be necessary for community workers to have open access to specialist hospital and community services, or at least open access to a full assessment without requiring a GP referral.

*"The CMHT nurse is only in the office once a week. I have to go to them even if I need visiting."*

*"There's nobody to get in touch with after office hours."*

*"Meetings are taking up all the CPN's time. Attitudes haven't changed."*

*Quotes from users*

- Access to rehabilitation services for serious mental illness and also for drug and alcohol problems should be easily available. Staff who work in these areas are encouraged to be willing to offer services to homeless people.

- Homeless people who are in contact with mental health services should have a full Care Programme and/or Care Plan if the client concerned is willing. Housing status should be included as part of all CPA assessments.

- Ward discharge procedures should include consideration of housing needs. The involvement of housing officers, working jointly with the clinicians who work with homeless people, to produce hospital discharge procedures will improve the service and also raise staff awareness of the problems.

- The staff of specialist mental health services should develop relationships with many groups of staff in facilities to which homeless people may go. The staff of hospital accident and emergency departments and general medical wards should be aware of the identities of mental health workers who have expertise, and they should be encouraged to make referrals of homeless people to the mental health service. There may be local GPs who offer a service to shelters or have clinics which people who are not registered with the practice may attend and they must have easy access to mental health services.

- The police are also likely to be points of contact, and local schemes for diversion from custody should be in place, with a ready access not only to inpatient beds but also to the whole range of community provision.

*"A day centre with walk-in clinical sessions is imperative, not only for homeless people but also for people in temporary bed and breakfast accommodation who will not be registered with a GP."*

Quote from user visitor report

## SKILLS

386   The health needs of homeless people are broad, and the age range of homeless users of specialist mental health services may also be wide. Specific skills are required to address problems such as those relating to drug and alcohol use and misuse, the recognition and assessment of major psychiatric disorders and an awareness of the problems of late adolescence.

*"The biggest help is other patients who have the time and ability to listen."*

*"A lot of people don't want help from the mental health services. Should this be forced on them?"*

Quotes from users

387   Specific kinds of understanding are required for work with homeless mentally ill people. For example, successful workers report that, initially, they are less active with clients, and spend more time listening in attempting to establish relationships before encouraging them to take up treatment. Counselling skills, as well as those of advocacy and those involved in developing long-term supportive relationships, may be of prime importance. The role of psychologists has been found to be very effective by some of the specialist teams working with homeless people.

388   Some skills may only be available from agencies outside the NHS, and workers should be willing to facilitate access to these for their patients. Examples include techniques for managing anger and violence, and helping male and female survivors of sexual abuse. They may be available from a number of agencies such as the probation services.

389 Skills in the assessment of risk both to others and to the client should be well developed. Specific components include the assessment of the risk of suicide, the risk of deliberate self-harm and the risk of violence. Further information on these clinical tasks is provided in *Suicide Prevention - The Challenge Confronted* (Williams and Morgan, 1994).

## PREVENTION

390 Well developed mental health services should aim to ensure that other systems of hospital and community care operate to prevent people with a mental health disorder from becoming homeless whenever feasible, and ensure that holes in the network of provision should be too small for individuals to fall through. Good case register systems are needed, which target high risk groups such as homeless people with enduring and/or serious illnesses and substance misuse problems. Not least, access to a wide range of appropriate housing, both supported and independent, will reduce the possibility that people with mental disorders may become homeless.

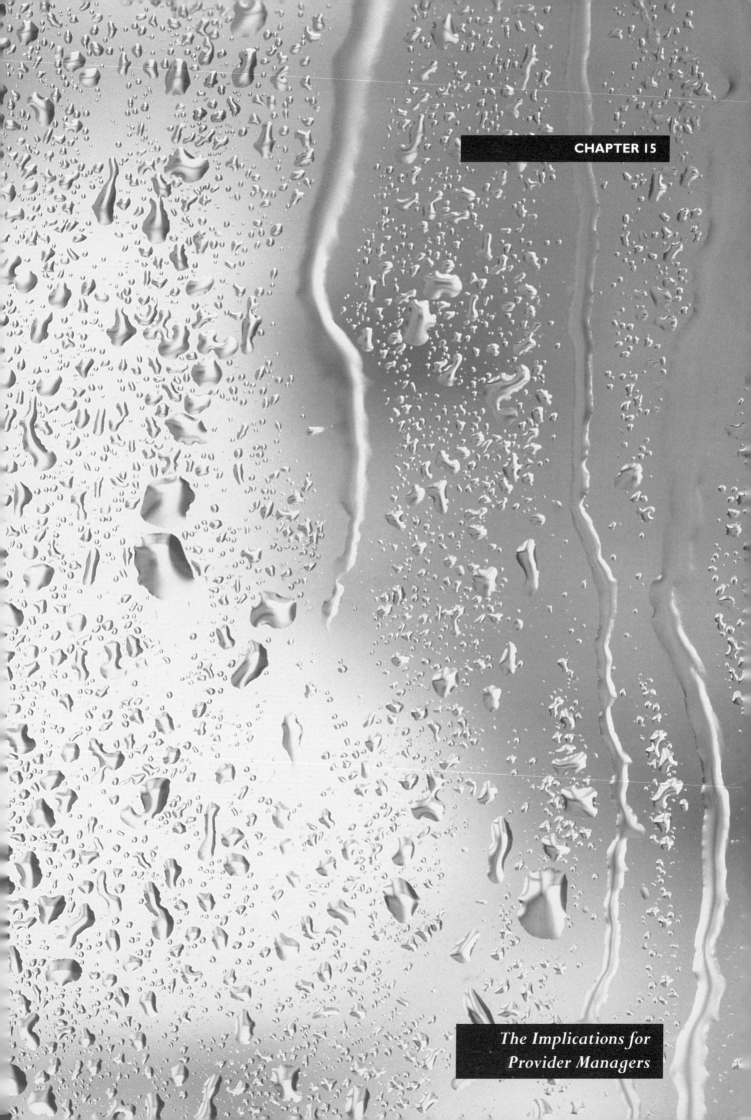

# CHAPTER 15

*The Implications for
Provider Managers*

## TRAINING

391 One of the significant findings of the service visits conducted by the HAS was the widespread lack of awareness at all levels of the issues concerning homelessness and mental illness. If access to services is to be improved, there are important implications for the training required by the managers of health services and that required by a wide range of professional staff.

392 The need for training applies at all levels, both for those service providers who do come into contact with homeless mentally ill people, such as those of accident and emergency units, and for those who generally see very few, for example, the staff of some primary health care teams.

393 The issues themselves are wide ranging and include:

- Background information on the local homelessness situation.

- Reasons for homelessness and the legislation relating to homelessness.

- The effects of homelessness on health, and more detailed consideration of vulnerability to particular illnesses which may be present simultaneously, eg schizophrenia, tuberculosis and foot problems.

- The patterns of alcohol and substance misuse and the resulting health problems.

- The barriers to access to services commonly experienced by homeless people. This is a key matter, which includes issues affecting GP registration, discrimination, prejudice and lack of information.

- Use of accident and emergency services and responses of their staff to homeless people.

- The perceptions of homeless people of their actual problems compared with common stereotypes.

- Service monitoring - recording housing status, tracking systems.

- Community services available to homeless people - processes of networking with voluntary agencies, housing associations and other providers.

- Sub-contracting with voluntary organisations.

- Care planning for homeless mentally ill people.

- Preventing professional isolation - eg the staff of chest clinics, sexual abuse workers.

394 As an example of good practice, the training programme on homelessness, provided by North East Thames Regional Health Authority in 1993, gave comprehensive coverage to all the issues listed above.

395 There are considerable benefits to clients and staff if part of any training programme is organised on a cross-agency basis, thereby pooling resources and expertise. General background presentations on health needs, vulnerability and patterns of homelessness could benefit any, or all, of the following services if they participate in shared training events.

- **Primary Health Care Teams**
  Fundholding and non-fundholding GPs
  Practice managers, nurses, health visitors etc

• **Acute Hospital Services (general)**
Accident and emergency, casualty units, and acute admission wards

• **Acute Mental Health and Psychiatric Services**
Crisis intervention teams
Psychiatric admission/acute wards
Day hospitals
Community mental health teams
Alcohol and drug problem services, including those which provide de-toxification

• **Social Services Departments**
Specialist mental health social work teams (including Approved Social Workers)
Generic social work teams
Occupational therapy services
Care managers/assessment officers
Welfare rights advisers/advocacy services

• **Local Authority Housing Departments**
Homeless persons sections/units
Hostel staff
Housing officers

• **The Non-statutory Housing Sector**
Housing association managers
Housing project staff

• **Other Agencies**
The Police
Probation services
Voluntary mental health organisations
Voluntary organisations that work with homeless people

396 In other circumstances, training may be more appropriately targeted at specific services. This may be because there are particular clinical issues, problems of access, or new information technology requirements.

*"The voluntary sector has enormous expertise in this area; insufficient use is made of that in the training of mental health professionals, eg nurses, social workers, medical students, junior doctors etc.".*

*Quote from user visitor report*

397 Staff who work directly with homeless people, and who have accumulated extensive knowledge and experience of the needs of their clients, are potentially very valuable contributors to specialist and general training programmes. So too are people who have experienced, or have attempted to gain access to, services. Training managers are strongly recommended to incorporate this expertise and first-hand experience into their training programmes.

## KEY ISSUES IN THE PROVISION OF SERVICES

398 Many aspects of the organisation and delivery of the care and treatment of homeless mentally ill people will be similar to those appropriate to the general population. However, the particular needs of this vulnerable group of people which have implications for service provision should not be overlooked. Account should be taken of the need to provide effective services for homeless people in the policy and practice of all aspects of NHS mental health and other health services. The matters covered below

are not exclusive but highlight key aspects of policy and practice which the managers of NHS provider units should ensure are in place for homeless people, in order to secure best practice.

- **The Care Programme Approach (CPA)**

  The introduction of the CPA, together with duties arising from Section 117 of the Mental Health Act 1983, and the introduction of supervision registers, are the key components of discharge planning which is intended to ensure continuing aftercare for the users of specialist mental health services. The CPA should be a basic tool for mental health services in their delivery of effective and efficient services that reduce the possibility of severely mentally ill people being lost to care. Practical procedures, which arise from these requirements, should address specifically the needs of homeless people as they may pose challenges to the provision of accommodation upon discharge and to maintaining continuity of care afterwards. As an example of good practice, the application of the Care Programme Approach by the Bath Mental Health Care Trust ensures that people are not discharged from hospital until appropriate accommodation, with some security of tenure, is available.

- **Community Mental Health Teams**

  The provision of specialist mental health services in the community is centred upon the work of community mental health teams (CMHTs) in very many places now. In order that the needs of homeless mentally ill people are met, it is essential that they have access to the services of CMHTs. This may require the staff of CMHTs with a general role to learn particular skills from the staff of specialist services for homeless mentally ill people. Other implications for CMHTs are that they may need to provide services in places to which homeless people go without issuing formal appointments.

- **Specialist Services**

  The provision of services by specialist teams or by individual members of those teams to homeless mentally ill people should not exclude their use of any other appropriate specialist mental health service. Specialist resources should facilitate referrals of homeless people to mainstream services, where and when appropriate, as well as acting as a resource to training mainstream services and as initial contact points for homeless mentally ill people. The HHELP Team in East London and the City incorporates all of these aspects of practice.

- **Relationships between the Providers of Primary and Secondary Care**

  Good relationships between primary care and specialist services are vital to the provision of comprehensive community-orientated mental health services. The ability to respond to the needs of homeless mentally ill people should be included in the range of tasks of community mental health services. GPs may need support and consultation if they are to take on more homeless people. In particular, GPs who attempt to meet the health needs of homeless people in a primary health care setting should not be disadvantaged by those patients having different levels of access to specialist secondary care advice when compared to people who have reliable accommodation. The managers and clinical staff of specialist services are encouraged to develop practices which ensure that GPs receive the support they need.

### · Information Systems

In the programmes of development and improvement of information systems to support their service and enhance care for users, NHS managers should maintain their awareness of the needs of homeless mentally ill people. Care for transient groups is likely to be enhanced by staff having easy access to information at the point of contact of patients with services. This might take the form of computerised record and information systems or of user-held records, as in a trial in East London and the City (Reuler and Balazs, 1991).

## LINKS WITH THE SOCIAL SERVICES DEPARTMENTS

399  Social services departments, as the leading agencies responsible for care in the community, should link with health services at every stage of service design and delivery. This includes collaboration in needs assessment, strategy, purchasing, service delivery and monitoring. Not only are the links between social services departments and health commissioners and also between them and providers pivotal, but their place within the range of local authority departments often provides them with the opportunity to act as a bridge to housing services. Their operational links with voluntary sector providers, through contracting and the allocation of Mental Illness Specific Grant and other ring-fenced grants, also give social services departments a key strategic position.

400  Matters of concern to the health service and local authorities can be raised at joint consultative and chief officers' meetings, and other joint planning forums. Surveys of need and service resource mapping can be jointly commissioned. Even if joint commissioning does not take place, health and social services can decide together which services are appropriately delivered by which agency, and draw up service specifications accordingly, if they share a joint strategy and share information on need and services provided. Agreement on common processes for ensuring the quality of data collection is also an important asset.

401  Some of the linking mechanisms are predictable. The inclusion of local authority social workers, resettlement workers and occupational therapists in providing multi-disciplinary services for homeless people clearly enlarges the effectiveness and accessibility of care. In new developments, such as court diversion schemes, collaboration with social services - as well as with probation officers, the police and court officials - in providing a multi-agency service for mentally disordered offenders is likely to have a beneficial outcome, since many service users are homeless people who have been charged with petty offences, often related to drink and drugs.

402  Social service departments may be willing to delegate their responsibilities and powers for conducting assessments and some of their purchasing functions to jointly composed specialist agencies in the statutory or voluntary sector. There are examples of such practice in Tower Hamlets. They facilitate the process of fast-track assessments which are often required by this client group.

**403** Similarly, the involvement of social services staff in designing and enacting discharge plans co-ordinated by the Care Programme Approach or in pursuit of the requirements of Section 117 of the Mental Health Act 1983 is necessary and desirable at all times. This is especially the case for mentally ill people whose needs are likely to be complex and challenging. Experience shows that joint work, involving hospital-based social workers, is often insufficient and that more formal links between health service personnel and area managers or senior care managers in the social services departments are also required to co-ordinate the provision of local authority services.

## LINKS WITH HOUSING DEPARTMENTS

**404** Throughout this report, reference is made to the importance of close working links with housing services. This section attempts to pull together the different ways in which mutually effective relationships can be established, with the aim of enabling homeless mentally ill patients to receive an appropriate mix of support services.

**405** A recent report entitled *Housing and Homelessness*, published jointly by the Department of Health and the Department of the Environment in November 1994, examined the *"interface and co-operation between housing, health and social service agencies in the provision of community care"* and *"the manner in which the community care needs of people with no settled residence were being addressed."* The findings of that report correspond very closely to the findings of the HAS visiting teams. This section draws much from that document.

**406** This report followed an earlier joint Department Circular of 24 September 1992 which recognised that *"adequate housing has a major part to play in community care"* and it called upon *"housing authorities to play a full part, working together with social services departments and health authorities so that each can effectively discharge their responsibilities."*

**407** Making this happen requires positive action by all three authorities. The development of a shared vision and strategy for community care and housing should underpin tripartite work. The active support for such a joint approach from the most senior managers and elected members of authorities is essential. Joint planning should be structured so as to enable full involvement by housing authorities.

**408** In the absence of collaboration of this kind, fragmented development is likely to persist. At present, it appears that many social services departments work with voluntary organisations, housing departments work with housing associations while health authorities are primarily concerned with re-provision plans for resettling people from long-stay hospitals. In this shifting patchwork of activity, homeless people may fail to receive either support services or housing. A co-ordinated strategy for developing housing alongside care provision would include use of options for involving a range of housing sectors, i.e. special needs and ordinary housing associations, local authority housing stock and other private and not-for-profit services.

**409** Joint planning groups should have a clear understanding of the cultural and operational differences between their agencies. They should have access to pooled information on each other's structural frameworks, planning and committee cycles and processes, as well as knowledge of the current and future available resources. This should enable, for example, epidemiological data to be considered alongside analyses of housing needs.

410 Once a joint strategic approach has been achieved, there are a number of ways in which effective collaboration can continue and these are summarised here. Responsibility for some of these possible initiatives may lie with one agency, whereas, in other cases, the identity of the initiating agency is less important than ensuring that action is taken.

### Lead Managers

Lead managers in social services departments could be designated, to take responsibility for co-ordinating policy and practice on housing and community care.

### Shared Posts

Suffolk County Council is cited in the DoH/DoE report (para 405) as having made a joint appointment at a senior level of a community care/housing development officer. This has proved highly effective in reinforcing existing good working relationships between the health, housing and social services.

### Joint Training

Training across agency boundaries at all levels, from senior management to the front-line level, is another important way of reducing single departmental approaches to providing services for homeless people with mental health problems and disorders.

411 In areas where housing and social services are organised on a unitary basis, there is likely to be a shared understanding of the constraints and processes affecting each service. Examples include agreement on the definition of vulnerability, and on care in the community policy.

### Joint Assessments

Several processes are possible in pursuing mechanisms for collaborative assessment. There is considerable scope for: merging assessments required by the care in the community policy with those conducted in pursuit of the Care Programme Approach with respect to hospital discharges; inviting housing staff to participate; and integrating care in the community assessments with housing assessments for homeless people. There are examples of these joint assessment procedures in the London Boroughs of Camden and Barnet, which have been facilitated by establishing joint vulnerability or mental health panels.

*One voluntary sector team visited by an HAS visiting team has been contracted to undertake community care assessments, and has been recognised by the SSI for its ability to fast-track assessments because of its familiarity with the user group.*

412 Fast-track referrals and assessment systems can be developed, which involve social services, health trusts, GPs and the housing departments, working alongside specialist staff who provide services for homeless people. An alternative mechanism could be that of the agencies agreeing to delegate a purchasing budget and powers of assessment and care management to certain specialist agencies.

### Joint Management of Housing and Care Support

Where services have been allowed to evolve in a fragmented way, inappropriate expectations can be held of housing managers. In these circumstances, they may find themselves responsible for people with high levels of dependency and needs which cannot reasonably be met by people who do not have necessary care skills. A joint strategy, which encompasses the provision of housing for people with a range of needs, should pave the way for the delivery of appropriate care to residents and tenants, and for the necessary training and support for housing staff by mental health workers. Some housing authorities interviewed in the HAS service visits complained that their willingness to allocate housing was not matched by the necessary level of treatment and social care from health and social services. The practice of employing peripatetic support workers, allocating community psychiatric nurses to individuals and ensuring the registration of patients with GPs, is especially useful as it recognises the multiple needs of vulnerable people in a flexible and cost-effective way.

413    The joint departmental report cited earlier found little evidence of co-ordinated commissioning strategies, and the authors attributed this to a number of causes. These included: lack of a common system of information about provision across agencies; complicated and unco-ordinated resource bidding processes which were seldom based on assessed need; and ineffective use of new technology. However, the report did highlight the circumstances in Nottingham where a concerted approach to funding by the social services department, health authority, FHSA and a Department of the Environment grant to the voluntary sector has resulted in exemplary community service for homeless people. The HAS visiting team which visited this service was impressed by its organisation. One thousand four hundred temporary bed spaces for homeless people are provided by the 40 member organisations of the Hostels Liaison Group. This group provides advice, training, information and a consultancy service. Assessments and fast-track admissions are organised by the multi-disciplinary mental health support team. One thousand referrals are handled annually. The level of co-operation between the different agencies has transcended the structural difficulties which, elsewhere, are impeding joint commissioning. This model offers a useful and tested approach to collaborative cross-sectoral service provision.

414    In the London Borough of Camden, housing services are fully integrated into the process of joint commissioning and the assistant director of the housing department is a joint commissioner. In this way, the housing department contributes to setting local priorities for community care.

415    One result of this approach is a community support pilot scheme which will provide various levels of support for single people who have mental health problems. Two voluntary organisations, one with a track record of developing housing for people leaving psychiatric hospitals, and the other that works with homeless people in the area, have been commissioned to develop this scheme. The key to the service is that it will provide individually tailored care, seven days a week (including evenings), which is flexible in type, timing and care. The scheme will be aimed at people at risk of losing their tenancies but there is flexibility for staff to begin by supporting people in bed and breakfast or hostel accommodation to help to sustain them through the period while they are waiting for a permanent tenancy. In the first year, the service plans to support 75 tenants.

416 The housing department has also transferred the management of one of its hostels for people with mental health problems, who do not wish to live alone, to a voluntary organisation working with people with mental health problems. This has enabled it to put money from the Special Transitional Grant (STG) into the hostel and so to provide the higher level of support which had been identified as needed by the tenants. This transfer has also enhanced the level of funding that is available for recreational and social purposes, raised the level of resident participation in the project, and ensured that more appropriate levels of support are available.

417 Another area of development in Camden is that of joint training. The Joint Training Forum has representatives of the health, housing and social services. Training officers from each have developed joint training programmes on community care. Each department has a commitment to sending equal numbers of staff to these programmes.

418 The housing department in Camden has also developed a new community care post. The holder, among other duties, liaises with hospital staff over patients who are to be discharged, represents the department on the vulnerability panel, and provides training on homelessness to staff in hospitals. Every single homeless person accepted as a priority by the homeless persons section is referred to the housing support team which is part of the housing department. The team members are trained as community care assessors so there is a direct link between vulnerability assessments and community care assessments for those people who need this extra level of support.

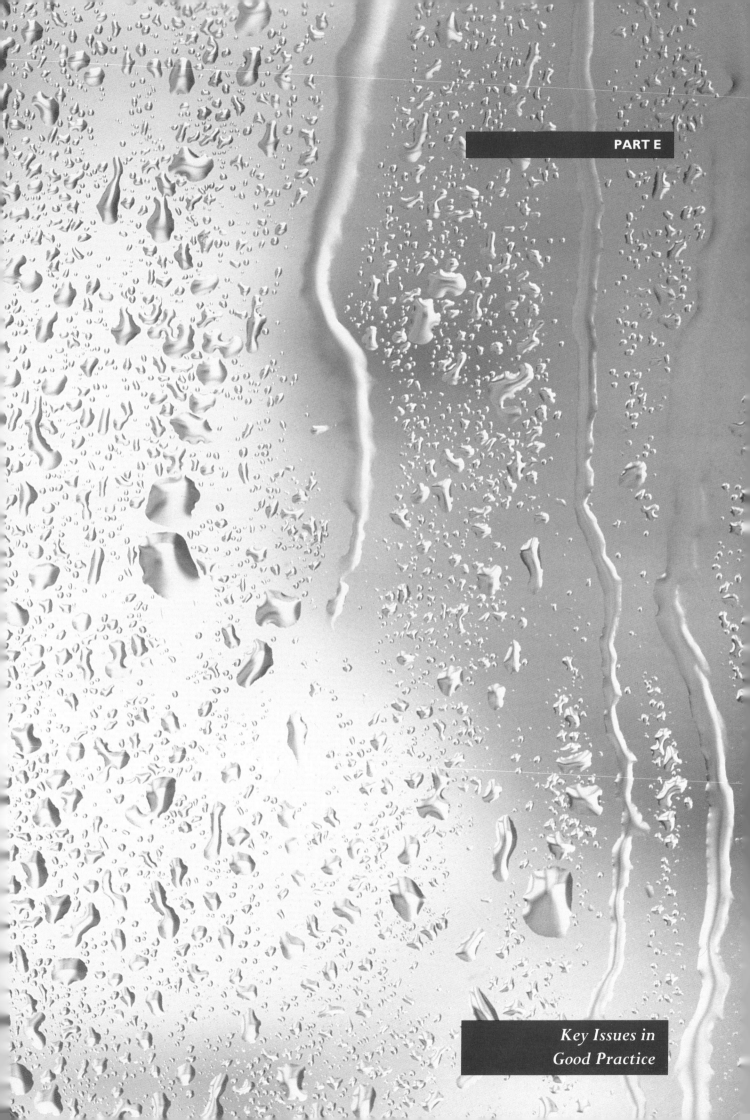

PART E

Key Issues in
Good Practice

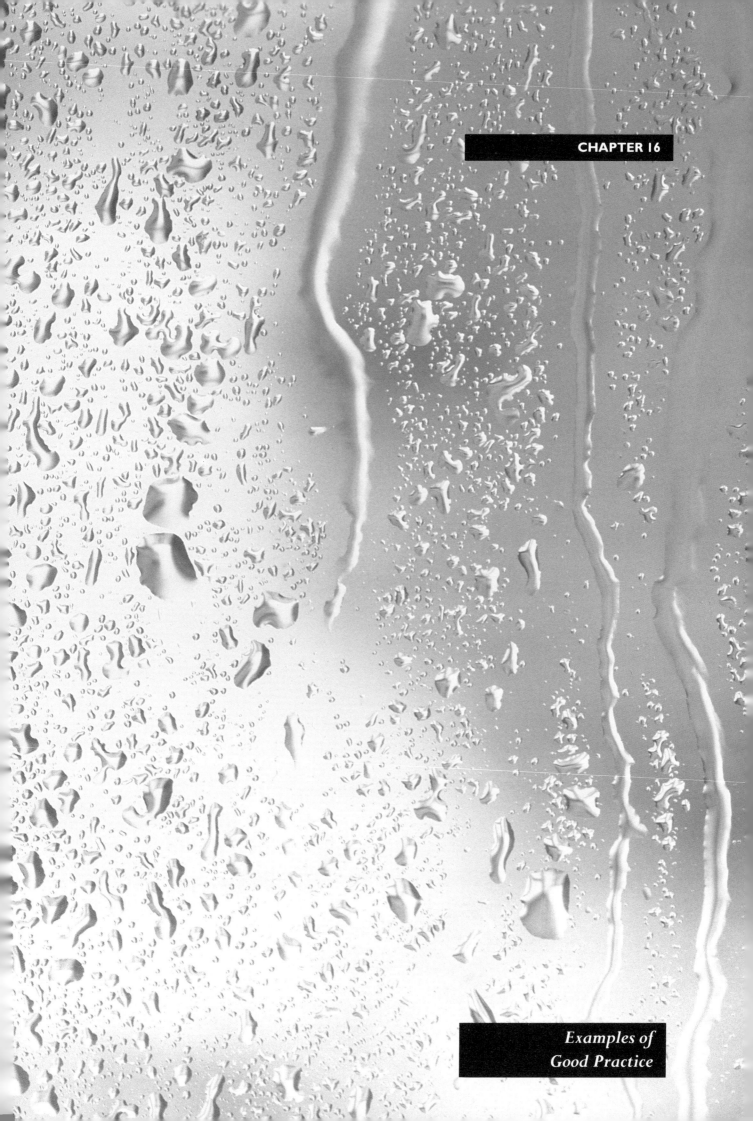

# CHAPTER 16

*Examples of
Good Practice*

## INTRODUCTION

419 The fieldwork for this review has enabled the HAS to identify a range of good practices in the commissioning and delivery of care to homeless people with mental health problems and disorders.

420 Some of the examples of good practice are ones which have universal value, and these could be put into effect in any service. Other examples demonstrate a creative response to particular local circumstances. Some might be helpful to, say, a seaside resort with a large number of bed and breakfast establishments, while other examples might be appropriate to rural areas. In a break from our traditional approach in reporting thematic reviews, we refer to particular authorities, trusts and locations, reflecting the importance of this geographical factor.

421 The HAS is aware that some outstandingly good practice has been made possible by an injection of additional capital and revenue resources by central Government. To expect authorities to achieve similar results without such a financial advantage might not be reasonable, yet the HAS did identify some very impressive work elsewhere. To an extent, identification of this latter group of good practices has aided pinpointing those elements which contributed to good practice.

422 The examples of good practice which impressed the HAS visiting teams are set out under the following headings:

- Strategic and operational planning (including information systems, research and development initiatives and consultation)

- Individual care planning

- Primary health care

- Alcohol and drug misuse services

- Multi-agency work

- Long-term care

- Acute and emergency care

- User involvement and advocacy

- Service development

- Training

## STRATEGY

### North Yorkshire

423 North Yorkshire District Health Authority and FHSA have produced a joint *'Strategy for Health 1994-99'*. One of the 10 priority areas for health gain within that strategy is health care for homeless people. A section on the opportunities for health gain acknowledges that *"those who are roofless may have a higher incidence of drug misuse, alcohol misuse or mental illness, and services need to be tailored for this group."*

424 This strategy also includes five key actions for health gain:

- To raise awareness of the impact of homelessness on health care with primary care and accident and emergency staff;

- To develop a flexible means of registration of homeless people with general practitioners which does not depend on having a fixed address.

- To develop ways of distributing information to homeless people on how to gain access to health services.

- To define the responsibilities of health agencies in obtaining and providing health care for homeless people.

- To work with homeless people to develop further action with the relevant agencies in the county.

425 This part of the strategy was the result of consultation with user groups and the voluntary sector.

426 The strategy has subsequently been turned into an action plan to *"address the link between health and homelessness in North Yorkshire."*

427 Four factors were identified as having influenced strategy development on homelessness:

- Heightened awareness, due to the increasing number of people sleeping on the streets of York;

- Increasing emphasis from the Regional Health Authority following work by the Regional Director of Public Health and additional research;

- Increasing pressure from the voluntary sector through partnership groups;

- Commitment from staff in the FHSA to develop services in this area.

428 An early target was to create a shared, strategic framework within which to co-ordinate separate commissioning activities around common goals. For the purposes of this report the relevant priority areas for development agreed by the Strategic Joint Commissioning Forum in January 1994 included:

- Drugs, alcohol and substance abuse

- Homelessness

- Crisis intervention for people with mental health problems

- Development in advocacy services

429 Each of these areas, together with other priority areas, will be developed by a task group at either county or local level and will be presented in the form of:

- agreed strategies to deliver specified outcomes;

- a critical path for further work and targets;

- a commitment to future resource allocation either from growth or replacing current service provision. The reports will provide the information base from which the Strategic Commissioning Forum will identify and prioritise the 1995-96 commissioning programme.

**430** In order to inform and co-ordinate knowledge of specific need, partnership groups have been set up in each locality. These are multi-agency groups with representatives from voluntary sector agencies, the health service, social services and from user groups.

**431** Members of the partnership groups have particular knowledge of the needs in their locality and areas of need highlighted by them included those of homeless people and those of people experiencing mental illness. This information was fed back to the planning co-ordination groups, and thence to the Strategic Commissioning Forum.

**432** As a result, special task groups were set up to correlate information on these areas of specific need. The task group concerned with homelessness is led by the housing department and consists of approximately 30 people, including GPs, and researchers from the University of York. Its report is due to be completed in September 1995. The report from the task group set up to monitor mental health issues and, more specifically, to monitor the effectiveness of the Care Programme Approach, is due in July 1995.

*Key learning point*

> The importance of creating a shared strategic framework within which to co-ordinate separate commissioning activities around common goals.

## Barnet

**433** Barnet Health Agency, the integrated commissioning body consisting of the District Health Authority and the FHSA, has begun work on a needs assessment for homeless mentally ill people and has included this as an issue to be addressed in its five-year strategy. There is a specific reference to the treatment of homeless people in Barnet Health Agency's specifications for adult mental health and accident and emergency services.

**434** Joint planning in Barnet has carried forward the strategy in a number of directions. This includes an imaginative use of the Mental Illness Specific Grant in relevant parts of the voluntary sector including its distribution to housing and providers of community care. At the time of the HAS fieldwork, the local authority was in the process of recruiting a homelessness link worker in order to improve access of those in need to mental health care.

*Key learning point*

> The importance of a systematic and comprehensive needs assessment so that services for the client group are included in local strategies.

## INDIVIDUAL CARE PLANNING

### Bath and Central Manchester

**435** In Bath and Central Manchester, the health agencies were able to demonstrate a commitment to making the Care Programme Approach more effective. While these efforts were targeted on patients awaiting hospital discharge, any improvement is likely to have a beneficial effect for homeless mentally ill people as well. The key to successful working of the CPA is good collaboration with social services departments, and this was the case in both the districts mentioned. In Central Manchester, a post has been created of co-ordinator of the Care Programme Approach to develop this joint work further. This co-ordinator has responsibility for developing a coherent operational policy aimed at fully involving all relevant agencies.

### East London and the City

*"The successes that are achieved with homeless people with long-term mental health problems are underpinned by having accessible and appropriate health care services in this locale."*

*Quote from user visitor report*

**436** In the area covered by this health authority, the specialist community mental health team (part of the HHELP Team) working with homeless people (and funded through the Homeless Mentally Ill Initiative) has been given delegated powers to carry out care assessments by the local authority and it has access to ring-fenced monies. Therefore the team also carries the responsibilities of care managers. The same authority, in partnership with the social services department, also delegates assessment and care purchasing responsibility, along with a budget from both the health and social services for alcohol and drugs treatment and care. These responsibilities are carried out by designated 'umbrella' agencies in the voluntary sector which sub-contract with other specialist agencies. At present, the division of purchaser and provider functions within the voluntary sector is also being formalised. The current and proposed arrangements are proving very effective in offering a speedy response to clients' needs and in providing a range of innovative services in accessible, non-stigmatising settings. It is important to note that these measures do not require the allocation of any additional resources. Rather, experience indicates that the problem in making these arrangements is that they require some decisions to be made at member level in order to delegate spending powers to the non-statutory sector.

*Key learning point*

The impact of a designated co-ordinator for the Care Programme Approach.

The effectiveness of service delivery can be improved by delegating budgets and assessment powers to specialist agencies.

## PRIMARY HEALTH CARE

### East London and the City

437   This is also an area where homeless people have good access to GPs and other primary health care workers. The HHELP Team is funded by the Department of Health for 17 general practice sessions a week. This involves eight local GPs and represents 1.7 whole-time equivalents. The sessions are used flexibly. In some instances, GPs run surgeries in hostels and day centres. In others, they see homeless people in their ordinary surgeries, and operate a flexible policy about appointments and surgery hours. The payments for these sessions are made over and above the ordinary payments that the GPs can usually claim for sessional work, and they are therefore an incentive for staff who are already committed to this task. It is the view of the HHELP Team that this arrangement works better than the practice of having one salaried GP attached to the service, as it appears to promote easier access to mainstream services. At present, the Department of Health acts as the purchaser and it is not certain whether this responsibility will pass, with the money, to the local health authority.

438   Also available, as part of the range of primary health care services, are general nursing and chiropody services. There are arrangements in force for homeless people to have access to local opticians and further negotiations are in hand to fund a dentist to work specifically with homeless people.

### North Yorkshire

439   Here, the FHSA has taken an active role in ensuring that homeless people are registered with GPs. The FHSA's stated policy is that the lack of a permanent address should not be a barrier to registration. All the GPs in the area have received letters reiterating this policy and asking them whether they are prepared to offer registration to homeless people in their area. Fifty-two practices (46%) replied. The implementation of this policy is being systematically monitored, and training on issues of importance to homeless users being offered.

### Barnet

440   In Barnet, there is a health visitor who has designated responsibilities for tracking homeless families and ensuring that there are contacts between the health services in the area of origin and those of the host borough.

### Bath

441   Avon Health Commission (previously Avon FHSA), through funding from the Department of Health, has set up a multi-disciplinary primary health care team to work with homeless people in Bath. This team is able to provide care directly at a voluntary sector night shelter and at the day centre in Julian House. These services are provided in a church crypt by a small team of workers who appreciate greatly the input from the primary health care team, both in respect of the care it provides to clients and for the support it provides to the staff of the scheme.

*"There is no specific statutory provision for homeless people with mental health problems, no relevant service nor outreach work, neither did it appear that there are any plans for such a service in the near future ... There was one service which was geared directly to the immediate needs of homeless people..."*

*Quote from user visitor report*

442    While the cost of this team is currently met through Department of Health funding, it should be possible to provide services of this kind out of existing budgets through a flexible deployment of resources.

*Key learning point*

The role of the FHSA in promoting the registration of homeless people with GPs.

The employment of GPs, on a sessional basis (with co-ordination by one GP and possible enhanced payments), to work with homeless people.

## ALCOHOL AND DRUG MISUSE SERVICES

### Bath

443    In Bath, the Mental Health Care Trust sub-contracts with the Alcohol Advisory Service and the Bath Area Drugs Advisory Service for them to provide counselling and support including advisory and information services. Both agencies have contracts with the County of Avon Social Services Department for conducting community care assessments for people who misuse substances, including alcohol. At this level, the practice is excellent. However, it should be noted that both these voluntary sector agencies are very concerned about the long-term shortage of beds for detoxification and the length of the waiting list for appointments with the specialist consultant psychiatrist.

444    In the same area, there is an effective, sub-contracted needle and syringe exchange service, which is operated by Bath and District Drugs Advisory Service and funded by the Avon Health Commission.

### Bradford

445    There are several voluntary agencies in Bradford which meet a range of needs among people who have drug and alcohol problems. The Horton Housing Association provides a 10-bed residential care home for homeless men with long-term alcohol problems. It also provides six bedsit units for patients who are mentally ill. Additionally, this project has plans to develop further supported accommodation, in the form of eight beds and 10 supported flats.

446    A further example of good practice in Bradford is the Bridge Project. This is a 'street' drug and alcohol agency (which also runs a small hostel for 10 adults and eight children). It runs a needle exchange programme, provides condoms and safer sex advice. One GP practice has offered to help with methadone prescribing.

447    There are two further Bradford schemes: the Piccadilly Project, working with homeless people with alcohol problems, is trying to make its services more accessible to black and ethnic communities; Project 6 is a counselling and advice service for people with drug, alcohol and solvent misuse problems.

448    The spread and range of services of Bradford's voluntary sector alcohol and drug agencies suggest a concerted response to identified needs.

### Mid Glamorgan

449   Mid Glamorgan has a well developed statutory service for drug and alcohol treatment. There are eight satellite clinics in this district. This is an important arrangement because of the self-contained nature of the communities and the serious lack of transport services.

450   There is also a needle and syringe exchange scheme led by the Community Pharmacy Service.

451   A voluntary agency, DASH (Drug and Alcohol Self-Help), is worth mentioning as an exemplar of good practice because of its work with people who are not in touch with any other agency. DASH undertakes work with children as young as nine years old.

452   However, it should be noted that Mid Glamorgan has no beds for detoxification, and that serious concerns were expressed by local people about the high prescribing levels of minor tranquillisers.

*Key learning point*

> The accessibility of needle and syringe exchange services to homeless people.
>
> The lack of inpatient detoxification services in general, and/or for homeless people, in particular.

## MULTI-AGENCY WORK

### Barnet

453   The London Borough of Barnet's structure, in which its housing and social services are integrated into one directorate, clearly enables inter-agency work at all levels. In the case of homeless mentally ill people, this is exemplified: by the attachment of a social services occupational therapist to the homeless persons' section; by a health visitor with specific responsibility for working with both single people and homeless families; and by the multi-disciplinary panel, drawn from the health, social and housing services, which considers all applications for local authority housing. The creative use of the Mental Illness Specific Grant also indicates the effectiveness of collaboration with the voluntary sector in Barnet.

### Powys

454   In Powys, there is an innovative example of inter-agency work, in which a general practice in Brecon is introducing a Citizens Advice Bureau into the surgery. In another practice in the same area, there are monthly visits to the surgery from a staff member of the local Benefits Agency. Additionally, each general practice in Powys is linked to a named social worker and a named community psychiatric nurse.

*"The best and worst examples of care were found in the voluntary sector."*

455   In the Montgomery area of Powys, the links between housing services and the local community mental health team are well developed. An occupational therapist at Welshpool co-ordinates the Housing Initiative Group which meets monthly to discuss individual client's housing needs.

### East London and the City

456 The ethos and practice of the HHELP Team, in developing strong support to the staff of voluntary organisations, was identified as particularly helpful. During the service visit, reference was made to the way the HHELP Team enabled these agencies to develop, rather than dictating to them about how to care for their clients.

### Nottingham

457 In Nottingham, good co-ordination, planning and training has been achieved through the development of the Hostels Liaison Group which was set up in 1981. The Community Health Team for Homeless People provides good primary health care for both single homeless people and families and it has good relations with both the voluntary and statutory sector services.

*Key learning point*

The effectiveness of linking specifically identified staff from different agencies with each other's service.

The importance of the other health, local authority and voluntary sector services working closely with local authority housing services at all times and at all levels.

## LONG-TERM CARE

### Central Manchester

458 In the central sector of Manchester there is a community support team which works with 36 people who have enduring mental disorder. The team's main objective is that of reducing psychiatric hospital re-admission rates for this group.

### Blackpool, Wyre and Fylde

*"There is a need for more resources to provide services to homeless people now."*

*Quote from user*

459 The local authority, through Mental Illness Specific Grant funding, provides a community support team, which covers the whole district and which gives continuing support to people who live on their own or with relatives. These are people who have a long-term psychotic illness and who have not benefited from other interventions. A particular aspect of good practice is the reports made by the team on the measured outcomes which result from its work.

### Mid Glamorgan

460 The work of the resettlement team, which organises aftercare and accommodation for people with enduring mental illness, and the small drop-in service in Porthcawl for bed-sitter residents with enduring mental illness, are both seen as examples of good practice.

*Key learning point*

The importance of monitoring the effectiveness of the work done with people who have an enduring mental illness.

## ACUTE AND EMERGENCY CARE

### Blackpool, Wyre and Fylde

461 The main accident and emergency unit in the district is a busy department with 75,000 attendances per year. It handles the acute psychiatric emergencies which arise every day from the psychiatric unit and the community. This department was seen as impressive in that it undertakes regular audit of its activity. It has completed a specific audit of homeless attenders.

### Bradford

462 In the Casualty Department at Bradford Royal Infirmary, there is a home care co-ordinator. This is an innovative appointment with considerable potential if the services offered are applied to homeless people.

### Powys

463 The staff of the casualty unit at the Brecon Memorial Hospital adopt a positive and flexible approach towards travellers and other homeless people. They co-operate well with the nursing staff at the Mid-Wales Psychiatric Hospital at Talgarth, which is approximately five miles away, and transport and escorts between the two hospitals are provided.

### East London and the City

464 Considerable thought has gone into improving the accident and emergency services for homeless people provided at the Royal London Hospital. It is now policy to include registered mental nurses (RMNs) in the unit team, and for staff to work closely with the staff of the psychiatric ward on the same site. A directory of hostels and out-of-hours services for homeless people, together with guidance on access, is available to accident and emergency staff.

### North Yorkshire

465 The accident and emergency services at York District Hospital do not have a computerised record system. Staff have, however, compiled manual records of people who have identified themselves as being of no fixed abode, and of people whose primary diagnosis was a mental illness problem; also of those people falling into both groups.

*Key learning point*

The need to develop systems for recording housing status in accident and emergency departments.

The need for ready access to psychiatric assessment and services.

The need for information on resources and services for homeless people to be given to staff in accident and emergency departments.

## USER INVOLVEMENT AND ADVOCACY

### Mid Glamorgan

466     This authority has made consistent efforts to involve people with first-hand experience of using mental health services in the development of care. There are structures for consultation with users at all levels of planning. The local user groups, which have been developed and supported by the statutory sector, are well organised.

### Bradford

467     In Bradford, there is an active voluntary sector working with homeless and mentally ill people. The MIND group is largely made up of service users. The input of these organisations and of other service users to the Mental Health Forum, the Drug and Alcohol Misuse Forum and the Housing Forum, as well as their involvement in producing a policy on the Care Programme Approach, is clearly more than a cosmetic process.

### Blackpool, Wyre and Fylde

468     Action in Change is a group which has been set up by the Blackpool Council of Voluntary Service, with a view to ensuring users become part of the consultation process.

*Key learning point*

> The need to consider sensitive ways of involving service users in consultation, and feedback on the nature and quality of care provided.
>
> The need to be aware that not all voluntary organisations speak directly with the voices of service users.

## SERVICE DEVELOPMENT

### Nottingham

469     The work of the mental health support team, housed alongside the Hostels Liaison Group, in Nottingham is widely recognised as an example of excellent practice. The team's aims of improving the assessment and support of, and access to, mental health services for homeless people are being achieved through the work of experienced and committed professional staff.

### Powys

470     In Powys, two appointments have been made of development workers, one in the social services department and the other in the voluntary sector. The latter position is funded by the Welsh Office. These postholders, who work collaboratively, have been important in the strategy for the creation of new services and in the effective networking of mental health and other agencies across the country.

### Mid Glamorgan

471     A similar post within the Mid Glamorgan Association for Voluntary Organisations (MGAVO) has promoted imaginative work and increased collaboration across the voluntary sector and users' groups.

472 Another interesting and useful service is provided in a small social services residential unit for profoundly deaf people who have an enduring mental illness.

### Barnet

473 Barnet's use of the Mental Illness Specific Grant, to fund social services department fieldwork staff and to develop voluntary provision in the borough, has been very effective.

### North Yorkshire

474 The appointment of accommodation officers in each social services division has improved communication and referrals between the social services department, the housing department and the health service. The introduction of referrals panels has increased the choice and appropriateness of placements available to clients.

### Central Manchester

475 Overall, the work of the voluntary sector in the fields of housing and mental health is commendable in Manchester. The network of agencies which provide housing with support offers a degree of choice not often available elsewhere. Creative Support has appointed an outreach worker to develop a network for homeless mentally ill people. This is welcomed by users as accessible and because it is not part of the statutory services.

*Key learning point*

The effectiveness of appointing mental health development workers in both the statutory and voluntary sectors.

The inclusion of the needs of homeless mentally ill people when planning the distribution of the Mental Illness Specific Grant.

## TRAINING

### Nottingham

476 Training for their own staffs, and for other agencies, is seen as an important function by the Hostels Liaison Group and the mental health support team in Nottingham. Their work in this field is well thought out and developed and it has built upon the expertise of the staff, who have been able to raise awareness of homelessness issues within the statutory sector. They provide a range of training circuits and workshops locally, nationally and internationally.

*"In my view, a mental health team, such as that which is employed by Nottingham Hostels Liaison Group, is what is wanted."*

*Quote from user from another city*

*"Everybody mentioned the important work that the mental health support team does."*

*Quote from user visitor report*

**East London and the City**

**477**   In a similar way to the Nottingham team, workers at HHELP have also taken on a significant training function with regard to issues concerning homelessness. The training is targeted at staff working in general medical and mental health services, and in mental health issues for the front-line staff of hostels and day centres. This training function has served to raise the profile of street homelessness within mainstream services.

*Key learning point*

The recognition of the potential of the training resources which are located within specialist teams.

The value of harnessing locally available training expertise in service specifications with the intention of increasing the knowledge-base of commissioners and other providers.

# CHAPTER 17

*A Summary of Key
Concepts and Challenges*

## CONCEPTS

1  Homeless people are **not** a homogeneous group. The 'street person' stereotype probably represents no more than one in a hundred of the homeless population. Many of this population are hidden homeless. Up to 25% are female.

2  Homelessness is not just an **urban** phenomenon. The number of homeless people in **rural** areas is rising and is about 12% of the total homeless population nationally.

3  **Mental Illness** rates among homeless people are twice as high as those of the domiciled population, and are, generally, of a more severe nature. Disorders may be both a **cause** and a **consequence** of homelessness.

4  **Alcohol** and **drug misuse** is a significant problem for many homeless people. It may be present at the same time as a mental illness.

5  Homeless people often have **multiple** and **complex** needs. This may relate to multiple health problems as well as housing, social, financial and other problems.

6  The **priorities** of homeless people do not always put health care at the top of the list. Shelter, warmth, food and money may be ranked higher.

7  A significant proportion of homeless people have some contact with the criminal justice system. Recent studies show that twice as many of those with past or present psychiatric problems have been imprisoned compared to those without a history of mental illness. Crimes were largely against property and were alcohol-related.

## CHALLENGES

To gain information on the size, nature, location of homeless people in the area covered by the health authority.

To identify possible sources of information in other statutory and voluntary agencies.

To gain information on patterns of rural homelessness, including seasonal and migratory movements of homeless people; for example, of travellers and agricultural workers.

To undertake a needs assessment of the homeless population based on a comprehensive knowledge-base.

To incorporate this in the commissioning strategy for mental health and other relevant health services.

To ensure that there are close operational links between mental health services and the drug and alcohol advisory and misuse services.

To organise services in ways which allow for full assessment of individual needs in co-operation with other relevant services and agencies.

To undertake active health promotion targeted at homeless people, with accessible information on services.

To provide health care in settings which are used by homeless people.

To consider, in any commissioning strategy, how mentally disordered offenders can be diverted from the criminal justice system into appropriate mental health care. The police and the probation services should be involved in planning and consultation forums.

A SUMMARY OF KEY CONCEPTS AND CHALLENGES

| CONCEPTS | CHALLENGES |
|---|---|
| 8 The rate of **deliberate self-harm,** including **suicide,** may be seven times that of the general population. | To consider how the guidance in the HAS report *Suicide Prevention - The Challenge Confronted* and the Health of the Nation Mental Illness Key Area Handbook can best be applied in the case of homeless people. |
| 9 **Access** is the major issue in providing all kinds of health care for homeless people. Difficulty in gaining access may be due to: <br><br> - lack of information about local health services; <br> - lack of a permanent address; <br> - inflexible appointment systems; <br> - referral systems for specialist services which require registration with a GP; <br> - discrimination and prejudice; <br> - staff and users being unaware of this entitlement of homeless people to health care. | To inform homeless people about services. <br><br> To provide some services which accept self-referral. <br><br> To provide training for staff on making services more sensitive to the needs of homeless people. <br><br> To encourage GPs to provide health care for homeless people by full registration wherever possible. To consider ways of providing incentives to GPs to do this. <br><br> To develop out-reach services. |
| 10 Higher than average use is made of **accident and emergency services** by homeless people, largely because of the problems they experience in gaining access to primary and specialist mental health care. | To provide more accessible primary and specialist mental health services. <br><br> To achieve formal and effective liaison between accident and emergency departments and the agencies which work with homeless people. <br><br> To achieve formal and effective liaison between accident and emergency departments and with mental health services. <br><br> To ensure that monitoring of the work of accident and emergency departments includes collecting information on the housing status of attenders. <br><br> To provide information on services for homeless people to the staff of accident and emergency departments. |
| 11 Specially designated services for homeless people can improve **access,** but they may, at the same time, **marginalise** users and staff. | To ensure that specialist services for homeless people are planned and delivered in ways which promote contacts for both patients and staff with mainstream mental health services. <br><br> To consider both a short-term and longer-term strategies to overcome the dangers of marginalisation. |

| CONCEPTS | CHALLENGES |
|---|---|
| 12 Primary health care services offer the best level and setting for most care for homeless mentally ill people. | To consider how to develop primary health care services. |
| 13 "*Users* are also **experts.** *Most of them probably know better than anyone else what did help them, and what might have helped if it had been available. They also know what it feels like to be mentally ill and on the receiving end of care.*"<br><br>- *User of mental health services* | To develop a commitment to the involvement of past and present service users.<br><br>To promote and purchase advocacy and self-advocacy services.<br><br>To establish and support consultative machinery which involves users at all levels of strategic and operational planning. |
| 14 **Voluntary organisations** are the major providers of services for homeless people. Frequently, they also have useful information on the numbers of homeless people, their needs, and of the networks of other resources and agencies. | To develop healthy alliances with the voluntary sector.<br><br>To develop mature relationships with voluntary providers and enter into appropriate contractual processes with them. |
| 15 **Private sector providers** are seldom involved in consultation or regarded as contributing to collaborative partnerships. | To seek ways of involving bed and breakfast proprietors and other home owners in consultation and client reviews. To develop systems of accreditation for small establishments.<br><br>To liaise closely with local authority inspection and registration units. |
| 16 **Fragmentation of services** for homeless people can discourage an holistic response to their complex needs, and be a barrier to access. | To organise assessment, therapy, social support and care in an integrated way, using inter-agency and multi-disciplinary approaches. |
| 17 **Collaboration** between agencies, both commissioning and providing, at strategic and operational levels, will produce a more balanced and effective response to the needs of homeless people. | To ensure that there is maximum collaboration at all levels between health, social and housing services and the voluntary sector.<br><br>To have designated lead officers in each sector to co-ordinate collaborative work. |
| 18 A **shared vision** is needed to ensure effective collaboration. | To gain the commitment and support of health and local authority members, trust executive and non-executive directors and the senior managers of these organisations to joint working and, where appropriate, joint commissioning. |

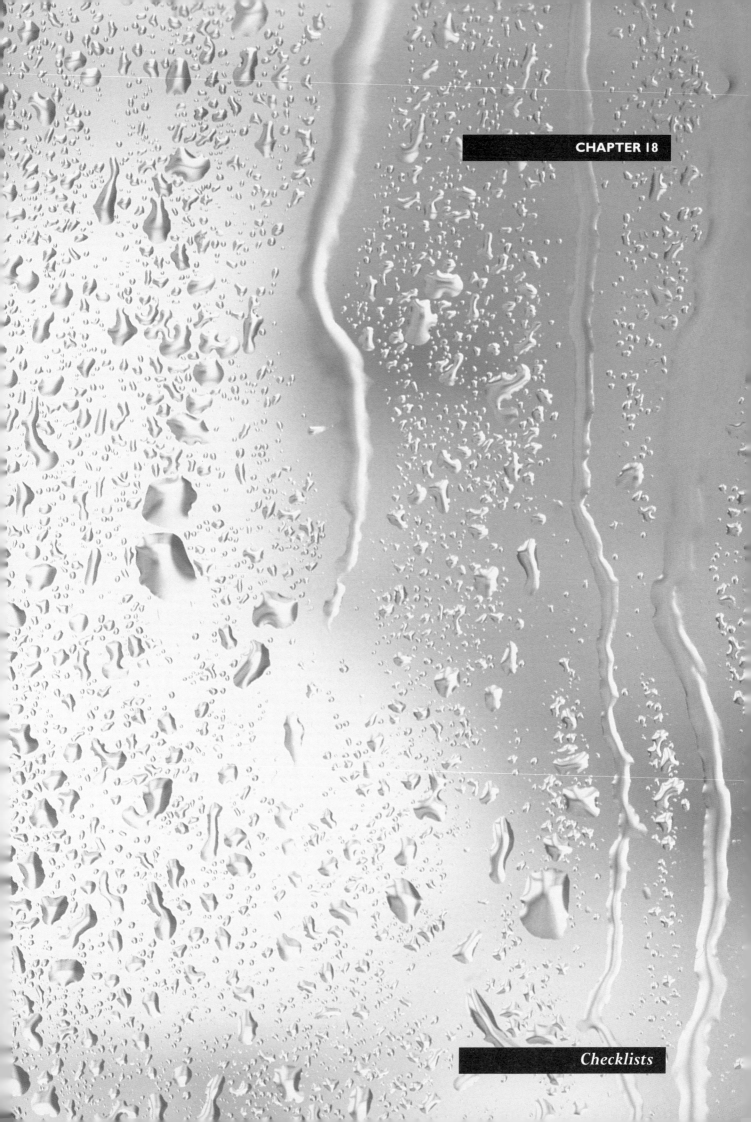

**CHAPTER 18**

*Checklists*

**This section contains some useful checklists which are drawn from the text of this report and tables within it. They are repeated here for easy reference.**

CHECKLISTS

## CHECKLIST 1

## THE THREE KEY GOALS FOR PURCHASERS

| |
|---|
| • Improve people's health by targeting resources on effective ways of delivering clinical care and promoting health |
| • Improve the quality of health care, making it more responsive to the wishes and needs of people |
| • Ensure that as many people as possible receive high quality care from what available resources can provide |

## CHECKLIST 2

## HEALTH OF THE NATION TARGETS FOR MENTAL ILLNESS

- To improve significantly the health and social functioning of mentally ill people.

- To reduce the overall suicide rate * by at least 15% by the year 2000 (from 11.1 per 100,000 population in 1990 to no more than 9.4).

- To reduce the suicide rate * of severely mentally ill people by at least 33% by the year 2000 (from the estimate of 15% to no more than 10%).

* Includes unexplained deaths

This checklist contains a selection of possible Health Gain And Service Targets taken from the Welsh Office NHS Directorate's *Protocol for Investment in Health Gain (Mental Health) April 1993'*. The following targets could usefully be applied to homeless mentally ill people.

## CHECKLIST 3

This checklist contains a selection of possible Health Gain And Service Targets taken from the Welsh Office NHS Directorate's *'Protocol for Investment in Health Gain (Mental Health) April 1993'*.
The following targets could usefully be applied to homeless mentally ill people.

| HEALTH GAIN TARGETS | SERVICE TARGETS |
|---|---|
| Reduce the suicide rate of severely mentally ill people by at least 33% by the year 2002. | NHS Commissioners and local authorities should develop good quality comprehensive, integrated local services to complement adequate hospital provision with appropriate levels of security by the year 2002. |
| Increase the proportion of those with a severe mental illness who have a permanent home with appropriate levels of support to 75% by 1997, and to 90% by 2002. | |
| Reduce the number of mentally disordered offenders who may be inappropriately placed within the Criminal Justice System and special hospitals to 10% by 1997 and less than 1% by 2002. | HAs, FHSAs, Probation Services and others should ensure that there are well developed and co-ordinated services/or the appropriate diversion of mentally disordered offenders from the Criminal Justice System by 1995. |
| Reduce the mortality rate from a physical illness for people with a severe mental illness by 10% by 1997 and by 20% by 2002. | Service specifications should ensure that: |
| Progressively increase social skills and support for people with a long-term severe mental illness. | -there is a co-ordinated approach to meeting the needs of those with a severe long-term mental illness by 1995 |
| | -those who need an individual care plan have one by 1995 |
| | -HAs, FHSAs, Social Services and others should ensure there are well developed and co-ordinated plans for the rehabilitation of people with long-term severe mental illness in the community by 1995 |

## CHECKLIST 4

## HOUSING ACT 1985 DEFINITIONS OF HOMELESSNESS

| People are considered to be homeless if they and those members of their family with whom they normally live: |
| --- |
| • have no accommodation that they are entitled to occupy; |
| • have a home but are unable to gain entry to it; |
| • have a home but are in danger of violence from someone living there; |
| • have accommodation which is moveable (for example, a caravan or houseboat) and they have nowhere to place it. |

**CHECKLIST 5**

**CATEGORIES OF HOMELESSNESS USED BY THE HAS**

| |
|---|
| • Street homeless people |
| • Travellers - New Age and traditional |
| • Single parents, including residents of refuges |
| • Refugees |
| • Homeless people from black and ethnic communities |
| • Homeless people in rural areas |
| • People in insecure accommodation, eg bed-sits, squats, friends' floors etc |
| • Psychiatric inpatients with no home to go to |
| • Homeless elderly people |

**CHECKLIST 6**

**MAJOR FINDINGS OF THE HAS SERVICE VISITS**

| |
|---|
| • Some instances of excellent or good practice (chapter 16) |
| • A low level of awareness of homelessness |
| • Lack of strategy in the commissioning and provision of services for homeless people |
| • Problems in obtaining the necessary information on homelessness and homeless people |
| • The strategic and operational importance of the voluntary sector |
| • Problems of access to services |
| • Problems in registration with GPs and the provision of primary health care services |
| • Challenges presented by mobile populations, ie travellers |
| • Difficulties in implementing the Care Programme Approach |
| • Underdeveloped local collaboration with housing services |

## CHECKLIST 7

## THE KEY PRINCIPLES OF GOOD PRACTICE

| |
|---|
| • Services should be offered on a drop-in basis with no appointment being necessary. Users should be able to refer themselves and be seen the same day if the need is urgent. |
| • An advocacy role should be central to the service offered to homeless people with mental health problems and illnesses. |
| • Work should be carried out in partnership between the statutory health and local authority services and the voluntary sector and community groups. |
| • Support should be provided to and through the services that people use. |
| • Mental health services should put more emphasis on listening and talking to homeless people prior to intervention. |
| • Community mental health services should be effectively publicised with potential users. |
| • Services should provide high quality clinical expertise, with evaluation of their effectiveness being an integral part of the work. |
| • Joint commissioning of services and multi-agency working. |
| • Diverse services for a diverse client group. |
| • Outreach work and out-of-hours services are important. |

**CHECKLIST 8**

**CONSIDERATIONS ON PROVIDING SERVICES FOR PEOPLE FROM BLACK AND ETHNIC GROUPS IN THE COMMUNITY**

| |
|---|
| • The composition of the staff employed should be developed to come to reflect the diverse cultural and ethnic make-up of the local area |
| • Ethnic monitoring |
| • Training for staff to help them to recognise and cater for the different cultural, religious and dietary requirements of their patients |
| • Availability of interpreters and translated information, including the provision of these services out-of-hours |
| • Availability of health advocates |

## CHECKLIST 9

## COMMISSIONING SERVICES

| The Seven Stepping Stones |
| --- |
| Good practice was highlighted by the service visits as falling into seven key areas for developing purchaser performance. The HAS service visits indicate that these conform well with the seven stepping stones in *Purchasing for Health.* |
| • Develop a multi-agency strategy |
| • Improve the knowledge-base of purchasing |
| • Effective contracts |
| • Increase responsiveness to local people |
| • Develop mature relations with providers |
| • Develop local alliances |
| • Improve the organisational capacity of purchasers |

| The Seven Imperatives for Effective Contracting Identified in Purchasing for Health |
| --- |
| • Better working between purchasers and providers |
| • Involvement of doctors in the contracting process |
| • Involvement of nurses in the contracting process |
| • Realism about activity and the impact of change |
| • Ensuring contracts are appropriate |
| • Effective monitoring arrangements |
| • Robust information on activity and prices |

| Seven Guiding Principles for Achieving Success in Purchasing Health Care |
| --- |
| • Listen to the service users |
| • Know what you wish to achieve |
| • Relate service contracts to targets |
| • Use information on effectiveness and outcomes |
| • Use contracts to engage providers in health promotion |
| • Use local clinical audit findings |
| • Establish challenging efficiency targets |

**CHECKLIST 10**

## An Idealised Approach to Commissioning Mental Health Services

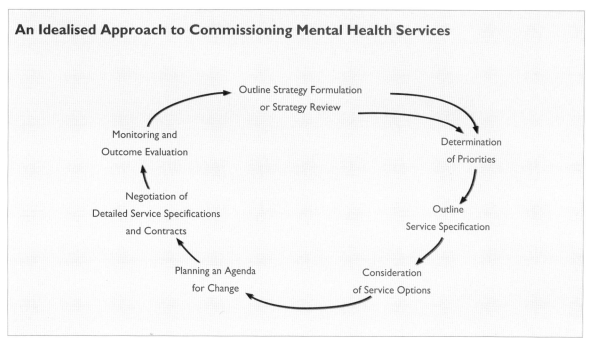

## Determination of Priorities

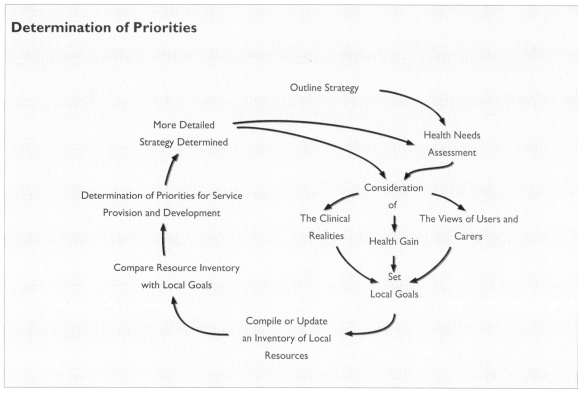

**CHECKLIST 11**

## THE KEY AREAS IN DEVELOPING A SOUND KNOWLEDGE-BASE

| |
|---|
| • A clear definition of the problem. |
| • Look to all sources of information. |
| • GP contact data. |
| • Local circumstances. |
| • The needs of the children of homeless people. |
| • Seasonal changes. |
| • Where are services currently being provided? |
| • Do all provider information systems record common data? |
| • What quality and audit systems are in existence?  Do any specifically impact on homeless people? |
| • Do the information and contract monitoring systems measure the access and take-up of the existing services? |
| • Is known epidemiological data being used in targeting service contracts? |
| • Do the training and attitudes of staff towards the problem affect service use? |
| • Are the views of service users taken into account? |
| • Is knowledge of known and effective interventions elsewhere available, and, if so, is it incorporated into service specifications? |
| • How are the contracts communicated to all those involved in their delivery? |
| • Are the service users aware of the service contracts? |
| • Do the results of information gathering inform future decisions? |

**CHECKLIST 12**

**THE NEEDS OF HOMELESS PEOPLE**

| An holistic approach should ensure that all the basic requirements of homeless people are considered. These include: |
| --- |
| • Somewhere to stay |
| • Something to eat |
| • Laundry facilities |
| • Health care |
| • Social care |
| • Access to more permanent housing |
| • Access to training, education and employment |
| • Access to recreation |

**CHECKLIST 13**

## LOCAL SOURCES OF INFORMATION

- Local authority social services departments
- Local authority homeless persons section
- General practitioners
- Voluntary organisations that work with homeless people
- Voluntary organisations that work with mentally ill people
- Health visitors
- Census returns
- The probation service
- Accident and emergency services
- Hostels
- Night shelters

**CHECKLIST 14**

**A SUGGESTED LIST OF CATEGORIES FOR MONITORING SELF-ASSIGNED HOUSING STATUS**

It is suggested that people seen in accident and emergency departments, psychiatric acute wards, and drug and alcohol advisory and treatment units be asked where they live and then given a list of accommodation types to choose from:

- Owned/rented flat/house

- Staying with friends, relatives or parents, by choice

- Staying with friends, relatives or parents against own wishes

- Local authority temporary accommodation

- Bed and breakfast hotel (DSS funded)

- Bed and breakfast hotel (as a tourist)

- Hostel

- Squat

- Night shelter

- Sleeping out

- Traveller

- Other (please specify)

## CHECKLIST 15

## CONSULTING SERVICE USERS

Consulting people who are homeless and have mental health problems is demanding. The first requirement is a commitment to respecting and taking seriously the views of homeless people who are experiencing mental health problems and illnesses. Developments may need to be taken slowly and in stages as involving service users requires sensitivity and flexibility. These are some ways of approaching the task.

- Health authorities could work with voluntary sector agencies and contract with those that work closely with homeless people to run discussion groups and find out about users' views on their behalf.

- Health authorities might contract for local research to be done on the needs of the homeless population and include users' views in the research specification.

- Health authorities could provide resources for local mental health users forums and ask them to carry out work on finding out the views of homeless users.

- Health authorities could ensure that patient satisfaction surveys carried out by providers take into account the fact that some people are homeless and ensure that surveys are sensitive to their interests. For instance, arrangements for monitoring patient satisfaction with Community Care Plans, care programming and discharge arrangements should always take into account the views of people who may not have their own home.

- Health authorities could include at least two service users on regular single-service or joint planning groups.

- Health authorities could appoint skilled advocates to liaise with users and feedback to statutory service commissioners.

**CHECKLIST 16**

**POTENTIAL PARTNERS IN LOCAL ALLIANCES**

- Drug and alcohol advisory and misuse agencies
- Social services departments
- District/borough housing departments
- Health authorities
- General practitioners and other primary health care staff
- Health service provider units
- Voluntary sector umbrella groups, eg Councils of Voluntary Service
- Probation service
- The Police
- Mental health voluntary agencies, eg MIND, National Schizophrenia Fellowship
- Local colleges and universities
- User groups - local and national
- Housing associations
- Churches
- Community Health Councils
- Residents and tenants associations
- Local press, radio, TV
- Private sector home owners

## CHECKLIST 17

## PARTNERSHIPS BETWEEN THE VOLUNTARY AND STATUTORY SECTOR

**What Statutory Purchasers and Providers Need to Know About Voluntary Organisations**

- Which client groups do they serve?
- Who runs them and what is their management structure?
- What are their aims and objectives?
- Who funds them?
- What services do they provide?
- What is their catchment area?
- Are they financially viable?
- How accessible are they to clients?
- Do they operate within an equal opportunities framework?
- What are the skills and qualifications of their staff?
- Are they familiar with contracting processes?
- Do the voluntary organisations have the capacity to expand?
- Do they attempt to involve service users in running their organisations?

**What Voluntary Organisations Need to Know as They Enter Into Partnerships with the Statutory Sector**

- Who are the key people in the statutory commissioning and providing agencies?
- What are their areas of responsibility?
- What are the commissioning and purchasing cycles?
- What arrangements are there for joint commissioning between the statutory health and social services?
- What kind of contracts are being negotiated  (eg, spot contracts, rolling contracts, yearly grants)?
- What kind of monitoring processes are required?
- Will core costs be recognised in contracts?
- Will training be available?
- Will any advocacy activities be in jeopardy?

**CHECKLIST 18**

**IMPORTANT CONTRACTING ISSUES**

| |
|---|
| • Targeted specialist approaches are effective in the short-term. |
| • GP and secondary care specialist staff should be involved in developing the overall strategy. |
| • Clinicians within both secondary and primary care should be engaged in advising on contract objectives and targets, audit, training and research. |
| • Locally generated information is likely to provide valuable insights, and specific incentives directed at practice level are also important. |
| • It is important to share the development of strategy, which is then linked to shared working, and, if possible, to joint funding and commissioning with other agencies (eg. social services and housing departments). |
| • There is considerable expertise in the non-statutory sector.  A mixed pattern of provision based on expertise and effectiveness is more successful than limiting purchasing to agreements with single agencies. |
| • Structure should always follow need, form should follow function.  Therefore local patterns of service may vary considerably. |

**CHECKLIST 19**

**ENSURING CONTRACTS ARE APPROPRIATE**

| | |
|---|---|
| The Access to Health guide on commissioning health services for homeless people sets out six areas for which targets and statements should be developed in all contracts. | |
| • **Access** | - Equity<br>- Staff attitudes<br>- Advocacy/interpreting<br>- Transport |
| • **Flexibility** | - Self-referral<br>- Appointment times<br>- Outreach work<br>- Hand-held records<br>- Multi-disciplinary approach |
| • **Training** | - For health staff<br>- For agencies that offer services to homeless people |
| • **Information** | - Provided at places to which homeless people go<br>- For staff about local services for homeless people |
| • **Monitoring and evaluation** | - Use of services by homeless people<br>- Outcomes for homeless users |
| • **Multi-agency work** | - Ensuring co-ordinated provision of services across agencies |

**CHECKLIST 20**

**MEETING PROVIDERS' EXPECTATIONS OF SERVICES**

- Develop a strategy which addresses better health, better health services and effective use of resources
- Ensuring financial stability of services
- Facilitating risk-sharing
- Having an explicit short-term agenda which is, preferably, shared
- Being willing to innovate and underwrite programmes of change
- Delivering what you say
- Being prepared to exchange information freely as between service providers for contracts
- Recognising that contracting is only part of the role
- Being sensitive in planning change and securing it
- Encouraging an approach to action planning that is based on continuous improvement
- Balancing recurring and non-recurring investments
- Encouraging excellence
- Realising that each relationship is different
- Expecting and anticipating changes in technical practice
- Expecting resources to be maximised - focus on the difference between delivery and maximising potential
- Encouraging providers to use their freedom

**CHECKLIST 21**

**POSSIBLE PERFORMANCE INDICATORS FOR MONITORING SERVICES FOR HOMELESS PEOPLE**

Apart from any other performance indicators that may be in place in mental health services, the following ones, if used consistently, should help to indicate the effectiveness of an agency in its work with homeless people.

- Definition of the target groups within the client population, eg street homeless people and/or those in short-term accommodation such as direct access hostels.

- Liaison with other agencies - especially primary care, specialist mental health, alcohol and drug advisory and misuse services.

- Written agreements or protocols, for access to psychiatric and medical advice and care.

- Agreed statements concerning the relationships between accident and emergency and other services.

- The level of work agreed for provision to people with alcohol and drug problems.

- An agreement to undertake assessments and to provide care in line with the Mental Health Act 1983.

- Estimates of the requirements placed on providers for their staff to be involved in the arrangements concerning housing and/or resettlement of homeless people.

- An agreement for statutory sector services to offer training to voluntary sector staff on care planning, health and housing issues.

**CHECKLIST 22**

**POSSIBLE QUALITY INDICATORS**

| |
|---|
| The quality indicators that are suggested here reflect both the intention to provide better access to services and the views of users on the need for an holistic approach. |
| • The ability of the provider to meet the requirements of The Patients' Charter. |
| • The effective operation of an open referral system. (Referral systems may be written or verbal and should be collaborative, involving the referrer, the service and the client.) |
| • The ability of specialist providers to complete a preliminary assessment within 48 hours of referral of all referred persons who are stated by their referrers to require this degree of urgent consideration. |
| • The allocation of a keyworker to clients where there is a need for longer term support. |
| • Regular (eg three-monthly) reviews of every patient. |
| • Evidence of an holistic approach to assessment and care. |
| • The operation of effective equal opportunities policies, including the provision of services that are non-discriminatory, and those that are sensitive to the needs of women, people from black and ethnic communities, disabled people, gay men and lesbians. |
| • Evidence of the operation of a system for consulting service users on their own care, and on service developments. |

## CHECKLIST 23

## A SUMMARY OF ADVICE TO COMMISSIONERS

| |
|---|
| • Establish a strategy that is shared with GPs, and which has a local focus. |
| • Share the strategy and encourage working with other agencies, especially local authority departments. |
| • Ensure contracts are negotiated which confirm and implement the strategy, and that the strategy is not led by contracting. |
| • Develop a clear view of the local context for commissioning and purchasing. |
| • Adopt a collaborative approach to contracting with providers, using explicit targets and risk-sharing. |
| • Encourage positive approaches to contracting, involving a mixed economy of providers from a range of sectors. |
| • Draw upon the views of users and voluntary agencies. |
| • Collaborate with clinicians on effective approaches. |
| • Consider positive incentives related to targeted work. |

**CHECKLIST 24**

**TRAINING – THE ISSUES**

- Background information on the local homelessness situation.

- Reasons for homelessness and the legislation relating to homelessness.

- The effects of homelessness on health, and more detailed consideration of vulnerability to particular illness, which may be present simultaneously, eg schizophrenia, tuberculosis and foot problems.

- The patterns of alcohol and substance misuse and the resulting health problems.

- The barriers to access. This is a key area that deals with GP registration, discrimination, prejudice and lack of information.

- Use of accident and emergency services and the responses of their staff to homeless people.

- The perceptions of homeless people - their actual problems versus the stereotypes.

- Monitoring services - recording housing status and tracking systems.

- Community services available to homeless people - processes of networking with voluntary agencies, housing associations and other providers.

- Sub-contracting with voluntary organisations.

- Care planning for homeless mentally ill people.

- Professional isolation, eg the staff of chest clinics, sexual abuse workers

**CHECKLIST 25**

**AGENCIES INVOLVED IN TRAINING**

Training needs are often best met through an inter-agency or inter-departmental approach. The following are some service provider units which relate to homeless mentally ill people, and may require training on homelessness issues.

- **Primary Health Care Teams**
  Fundholding and non-fundholding GPs
  Practice managers, nurses/health visitors etc

- **Acute Hospital Services (general)**
  Accident and emergency, casualty units, acute admission wards

- **Acute Mental Health and Psychiatric Services**
  Crisis intervention teams
  Psychiatric admission/acute wards
  Day hospitals
  Community mental health teams
  Alcohol and drug problem services including those which provide de-toxification

- **Social Services Departments**
  Specialist mental health social work teams (including Approved Social Workers)
  Generic social work teams
  Occupational therapy services
  Care managers/assessment officers
  Welfare rights, advisers/advocacy services

- **Local Authority Housing Departments**
  Homeless persons sections/units
  Hostel staff
  Housing officers

- **The Non-statutory Housing Sector**
  Housing association managers
  Housing project staff

- **Other Agencies**
  The Police
  Probation service
  Voluntary mental health organisations
  Voluntary organisations that work with homeless people

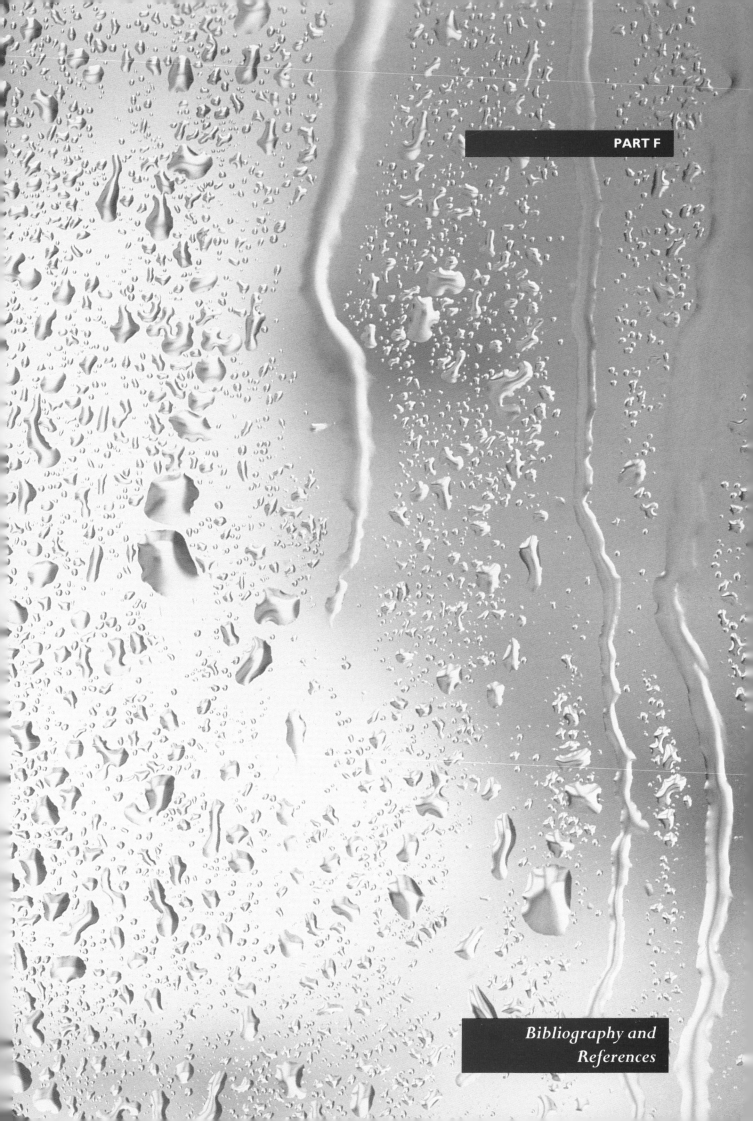

**PART F**

*Bibliography and
References*

# CHAPTER 19

## BIBLIOGRAPHY OF MAJOR RELEVANT LEGISLATION AND POLICY DOCUMENTS

*The Patients' Charter.* HMSO, December 1991 and 1995.

*The Health of the Nation.* HMSO, 1992 and 1994.

*The NHS and Community Care Act 1990.* HMSO.

*Developing and Weighting for Homeless People.* Access to Health, 1992.

*Purchasing and Poverty: A guide to Commissioning Health Services for Homeless People.* Access to Health, November 1992.

*Report of the Inquiry into London's Health Service, Medical, Education and Research.* HMSO, October 1992.

*Implementing Caring for People: Housing and Homelessness.* Department of Health and Department of the Environment. London, HMSO, 1994.

*Homelessness and Ill Health,* Royal College of Physicians. Lavenham, The Lavenham Press, 1994.

*Mental Illness - A Strategy for Wales.* Welsh Office, 1989.

*Protocol for Investment in Health Gain - Mental Health.* Welsh Office and Welsh Health Planning Forum, 1993.

*The Criminal Justice and Public Order Act 1994.* HMSO.

*Access to Local Authority and Housing Association Tenancies.* A Department of the Environment Green Paper. HMSO, January 1994.

## REFERENCES

**Access to Health, (1992).** *Developing an Age Profile for Five Homeless Populations.* London, Access to Health.

Access to Health, (1992). *Community Mental Health Services for Homeless People: Models of Good Practice.* London, Access to Health.

Access to Health, (1992). *Purchasing and Poverty.* London, Access to Health.

Alcohol, Drug Abuse and Mental Health Administration (1983). *Alcohol, Drug Abuse and Mental Health Problems of the Homeless.* Proceedings of a Round Table. Washington DC.

Alisky, J. M., and Iczkowski, B. A., (1990). *Barriers to Housing for Deinstitutionalised Psychiatric Patients.* Hospital and Community Psychiatry, 93-95.

Allen, I. and Jackson, N. (1994). *Health Care Needs and Services in Resettlement Units.* Policy Studies Institute.

Alstrom, C. H., Lindelius, R. and Salum, I., (1975). *Mortality Among Homeless Men.* British Journal of Addiction, 70, 245-252.

Arce, A. A., Tadlock, M. and Vergare, M. J. et al (1983). *A Psychiatric Profile of Street People Admitted to an Emergency Shelter.* Hospital and Community Psychiatry, 34, 812-817.

Arce, A. A., and Vergare, M. J., (1984). *Identifying and Characterising the Mentally Ill Among the Homeless,* p75-90. In The Homeless Mentally Ill, Ed: H. R. Lamb. Washington, American Psychiatric Association.

Austerberry, H. and Watson, S., (1986). *Housing and Homelessness.* London, Routledge & Kegan Paul.

Bachrach, L., (1984). *The Homeless Mentally Ill and the Mental Health Services*, p11-54. In The Homeless and Mentally Ill, Ed: H. R. Lamb. Washington DC, American Psychiatric Association.

Ball, F. L. and Havassy, E., (1984). *A Survey of the Problems and Needs of the Homeless Consumers of Acute Psychiatric Services.* Hospital and Community Psychiatry, 35, 917-921.

Barrow, S., and Lovell, A. M., (1982). *Evaluation of Project Reach Out 1981-2.* New York, New York State Psychiatric Institute.

Bassuk, E. L., (1984). *The Homeless Problem.* Scientific American, 6, 40-45.

Bassuk, E. L., (1990). *Who are the Homeless Families? Characteristics of Sheltered Mothers and Children.* Community Mental Health Journal, 26, 421-430.

Bassuk, E. L., Rubin, L. and Lauriat, A., (1984). *Is Homelessness a Mental Health Problem?* American Journal of Psychiatry, 141, 1546-1550.

Bassuk, E. L., Rubin, L. and Lauriat, A. S., (1986). *Characteristics of Sheltered Homeless Families.* American Journal of Public Health, 76, 1097-1102.

Baxter, E. and Hopper, K., (1982). *The New Mendicancy: Homeless in New York City.* American Journal of Orthopsychiatry, 52, 393-408.

Baxter, E. and Hopper, K., (1984a). *Troubled on the Streets: the Mentally Disabled Homeless Poor.* p49-55. In The Chronic Mental Patient, Ed: J. Talbott. New York, Grune and Stratton.

Baxter, E. and Hopper, K., (1984b). *Shelter and Housing for the Homeless Mentally Ill.* p103-139. In The Homeless Mentally Ill, Ed: H. R. Lamb. Washington DC, American Psychiatric Association.

Bennett, M. I., Gudeman, J., Jenkins, L., Brown, A., and Bennett, M. B., (1988). *The Value of Hospital Based Treatment for the Homeless Mentally Ill.* American Journal of Psychiatry, 145, 1273-1276.

Berry, C. and Orwin, A., (1966). *No Fixed Abode: a Survey of Mental Hospital Admission.* British Journal of Psychiatry, 112, 1019-1025.

Bines, W., (1994). *Health of Single Homeless People.* Centre for Housing Policy, University of York.

Birley, J., (1990). *Blame Homelessness, not the Hospitals.* Guardian. March 14, p21.

Blumberg, L., (1973). *What to Do About the Men on Skid Row; Report of the Greater Philadelphia Movement to the Redevelopment Authority of the City of Philadelphia.* Philadelphia, Greater Philadelphia Movement.

Breakey, W. R., Fischer, P. J. and Cowan, C. D., (1986). *Homeless People in Baltimore: Demographic Profile and Enumeration.* Paper presented at the Annual Meeting of the American Public Health Association, Las Vegas.

Breakey, W. R., (1987). *Recent Empirical Research on the Homeless Mentally Ill.* Paper presented at Alcohol, Drug Abuse and Mental Health Administration meeting on Research Methodologies concerning Homeless Persons. Bethesda, Maryland. July 13.

Breakey, W. R., (1987). *Treating the Homeless.* Alcohol Health and Research World, 11-42.

Breakey, W. R., (1991). *Mental Health Services for Homeless People.* In Homelessness: A National Perspective, Eds: M. Robertson and M. Greenblatt. New York, Plenum Publishing.

Brent Smith, H. and Dean, R., (1990). *Plugging the Gaps.* London, Lewisham and North Southwark Health Authority.

Brickner, P. W., (1984). *Medical Aspects of Homelessness,* p243-259. In The Homeless Mentally Ill, Ed: H. R. Lamb. Washington, American Psychiatric Association.

Brickner, P. W. and Kaufman, A., (1973). *Case Finding of Heart Disease in Homeless Men.* Bulletin of New York Academy of Medicine, 49, 475-484.

Brickner, C., MacFarlane, S., Paredes, R. et al, (1983). *The Homeless of Phoenix: Who are They? And What Should be Done?* Phoenix, Phoenix South Community Mental Health Centre.

Burt, M. R. and Cohen, B. E., (1989). *Differences Among Homeless Single Women, Women with Children, and Single Men.* Social Problems, 36, 508-524.

CARA, (1991). London. *Access to Housing for Irish Single Homeless People.*

Caton, C., (1990). *Solutions to the Homeless Problems,* p174-190. In Homeless in America, Ed: C. Caton. Oxford, Oxford University Press.

Caton, C., Wyatt, R. J., Grunberg, J. and Felix, A., (1990). *An Evaluation of a Mental Health Programme for Homeless Men.* American Journal of Psychiatry, 147, 286-287.

Central Statistics Office, (1989). *Social Trends 19.* London, HMSO.

*CHAR Advertisement,* (1988). New Society. January 15, p12.

Cohen, N. L., Putnum, J. F., and Sullivan, A. M., (1984). *The Mentally Ill Homeless: Isolation and Adaption.* Hospital and Community Psychiatry, 35, 922-924.

Corrigan, E. M., and Anderson, A. C., (1984). *Homeless Alcoholic Women on Skid Row.* Drug and Alcohol Abuse, 10, 534-549.

Crystal, S., Ladner, S., and Towber, R., (1986). *Multiple Impairment Patterns in the Mentally Ill Homeless.* International Journal of Mental Health, 14, 61-73.

Cumella, S., Williams, R. and Sang, R., (1995). *How Mental Health Services are Commissioned. The NHS Health Advisory Service Survey of Commissioners.* In Press.

Drake, M., O'Brien, M. and Biebuyck, R., (1982). *Single and Homeless.* Department of the Environment. London, HMSO.

Drake, R. E., Wallace, M. A. and Hoffman, J. S., (1989). *Housing Instability and Homeless Among After-Care Patients of an Urban State Hospital.* Hospital and Community Psychiatry, 40, 46-51.

Dreman, V. and Stearn, J., (1986). *Health Visitors and Homeless Families.* Health Visitor, 59, 340-342.

Eagle, P. F. and Caton, C. L. M., (1990). *Homeless and Mental Illness,* p59-75. In Homeless in America, Ed: C. Caton. Oxford, Oxford University Press.

Fernandez, J., (1984). *In Dublin's Fair City: The Mentally Ill of No Fixed Abode.* Bulletin of the Royal College of Psychiatrists, 12, 187-190.

Freeman, S., Formo, A., Alampur, A., and Sommers, A., (1979). *Psychiatric Disorder in a Skid-Row Mission Population.* Comprehensive Psychiatry, 32, 454-461.

Fischer, P. J. and Breakey, W. R., (1986). *Homelessness and Mental Health: An Overview.* International Journal of Mental Health, 14, 6-41.

Fischer, P., Shapiro, S., Breakey, W. R., Anthony, J., and Kramer, N., (1986). *Mental Health and Social Characteristics of the Homeless: A Survey of Mission Users.* American Journal of Public Health, 76, 519-523.

Gelberg, L., and Linn, L. S., (1988). *Social and Physical Health of Homeless Adults Previously Treated for Mental Health Problems.* Hospital and Community Psychiatry, 39, 510-516.

Goering, P., Paduchak, D. and Dubin, J., (1990). *Housing Homeless Women: A Consumer Preference Study.* Hospital and Community Psychiatry, 41, 790-794.

Goldberg, D. P., (1972). *GHQ The Detection of Psychiatric Illness by Questionnaire.* Oxford, Oxford University Press.

Goldfinger, S. M. and Chafetz, L., (1984). *Developing A Better Service Delivery System for the Homeless Mentally Ill,* p91-108. In The Homeless Mentally Ill, Ed: H. R. Lamb. Washington American Psychiatric Association.

Greve, J., et al (1986). *Homelessness in London.* GLC Research Team.

Grunberg, J., and Eagle, P. F., (1990). *Shelterisation: How the Homeless Adapt to Shelter Living.* Hospital and Community Psychiatry, 51, 521-525.

Hamid, W. A., and McCarthy, M., (1989). *Community Psychiatric Care for Homeless People in London.* Health Trends, 21, 67-68.

Harris, M., and Bachrach, L., (1990). *Perspectives on Homeless Mentally Ill Women.* Hospital and Community Psychiatry, 23, 253-254.

Health Visitors Association, (1989). *Homeless Families and their Health.* London, BMA Publishing.

Heptinstall, D., (1989). *Glimmer of Psychiatric Hope for Homeless Men in London.* Social Work Today, February 23, p16-17.

Herrman, H., McGorry, P., and Bennett, P., van Reil, R. and Singh, B., (1989). *Prevalence of Severe Mental Disorders in Disaffiliated and Homeless People in Inner Melbourne.* American Journal of Psychiatry, 146, 1179-1184.

Herzberg, J., (1987). *No Fixed Abode: A Comparison of Men and Women Admitted to an East London Psychiatric Hospital.* British Journal of Psychiatry, 150, 621-627.

Hinton, T., (1992). *Health and Homelessness in Hackney - Medical Campaign Project.* London.

Hinton, T., (1994). *Battling Through the Barriers - Action for Homeless People.* London.

Holden, C., (1986). *Homelessness: Experts Differ on Root Causes.* Science, 232, 569-570.

Hopper, K., Hamberg, J., (1986). *The Making of America's Homeless: From Skid Row to New Poor, 1945-1984.* Critical Perspectives on Housing. Philadelphia, Temple University Press.

Jones, B. E., (1986). *Treating the Homeless: Urban Psychiatry's Challenge.* Washington DC, American Psychiatric Press.

Kay, R., (1985). *The Homeless Mentally Ill.* US Department of Human Sciences. Vol.XI, Number 11, 6-9.

Kelly, J. T., (1985). *Trauma: With the Example of San Francisco's Shelter Programme,* p77-85. In Health Care of Homeless People, Eds: P. Brickner, L. Scharer, B. Conanan, A. Elvy, and M. Savarese. New York, Springer Verlag.

Koegal, P. and Burman, A., (1987). *Alcoholism Among Homeless Adults in the Inner City of Los Angeles.* Archives of General Psychiatry, 45, 1011-1018.

Koegel, P. and Burman, M., (1988). *The Prevalence of Specific Psychiatric Disorders Among Homeless Individuals in the Inner City of Los Angeles.* Archives of General Psychiatry, 45, 1085-1092.

Kroll, J., Carey, K., Hagedorn, D., Fire Dog, P., and Banvides, E., (1986). *A Survey of Homeless Adults in Urban Emergency Shelters.* Hospital and Community Psychiatry, 37, 283-286.

Lamb, R., (1984). *Deinstitutionalisation and the Homeless Mentally Ill.* In The Homeless Mentally Ill, Ed: R. Lamb. Washington DC, American Psychiatric Association.

Lamb, R., (1990). *Will We Save the Homeless Mentally Ill?* American Journal of Psychiatry, 147, 649-651.

Lamb, R. and Lamb, D., (1990). *Factors Contributing to Homelessness Among the Chronically and Severely Mentally Ill.* Hospital and Community Psychiatry, 41, 301-305.

Larew, B. I., (1980). *Strange Strangers: Serving Transients.* Social Casework, 63, 107-113.

Leach, J. and Wing, J., (1980). *Helping Destitute Men.* Tavistock, London.

Levine, I. S., (1984). *Service Programmes for the Homeless Mentally Ill.* p173-200. In The Homeless Mentally Ill, Ed: H. R. Lamb. Washington DC, American Psychiatric Association.

Linn, L., Gelberg, L. and Leake, B., (1990). *Substance Abuse and Mental Health Status of Homeless and Domiciled Low-Income Users of a Medical Clinic.* Hospital and Community Psychiatry, 41, 306-310.

Lipton, F. R., Nutt, S. and Sabatini, A., (1988). *Housing the Homeless Mentally Ill: A Longitudinal Study of a Treatment Approach.* Hospital and Community Psychiatry, 39, 40-45.

Lipton, F. and Sabatini, A., (1984). *Constructing Support Systems for Homeless Chronic Patients,* p153-172. In The Homeless Mentally Ill, Ed: H. R. Lamb. Washington DC, American Psychiatric Association.

Lowry, M. and Conlon, R., (1987). *The Homeless: Myths versus Reality.* Democratic Study Group, US House of Representatives, February, p1-7.

Lowry, S., (1989). *Health Needs of the Homeless.* British Medical Journal, 298, 771-772.

Lowry, S., (1990). *Housing and Health: Health and Homelessness.* British Medical Journal, 300, 32-34.

Maitra, A. K., (1982). *Dealing with the Disadvantaged - Single Homeless, Are We Doing Enough?* Public Health, 96, 141-144.

Mariasy, J., (1987). *Young People and Homelessness.* Everywoman, November, p12.

Marshall, E. J., (1990). *Psychiatric Morbidity in Homeless Women.* Paper presented at the Royal College of Psychiatrists Quarterly Meeting, Birmingham, July.

Marshall, E. J. and Reed, J., (1992). *Psychiatric Morbidity in Homeless Women.* British Journal of Psychiatry, 160, 761-768.

Marshall, M., (1989). *Collected and Neglected: Are Oxford Hostels for the Homeless Filling up with Disabled Psychiatric Patients?* British Medical Journal, 299, 706-709.

Matthews, P., (1986). *Doctors for the Homeless and Rootless.* British Medical Journal, 292, 1672-1674.

McCarthy, M., (1980). *London's Health Services in the 80s.* King's Fund Project Paper No 25.

McKechnie, S., (1988). *After Dark.* Channel 4, March 4.

Merves, E., (1986). *Conversations with Homeless Women.* Unpublished Doctors Dissertation. University of Minnesota, USA.

Morrisey, J. and Levine, I., (1987). *Researchers Discuss Latest Findings, Examine Needs of Homeless Mentally Ill Persons.* Hospital and Community Psychiatry, 38, 811-812.

Morse, G. and Calsyn, R., (1986). *Mentally Disturbed Homeless People in St Louis: Needy, Willing, But Underserved.* Journal of Mental Health, 14, 74-94.

Niven, P. and Thomas, A., (1989). *Living in Temporary Accommodation.* London, HMSO.

O'Neill, M., (1988). *Tunnel Vision.* Insight. September, p12-15.

O'Neill, M., (1989). *Users of Resettlement Units: A Report of a Survey Carried out in Fifteen Resettlement Units and Census Carried Out in all Twenty-Two.* London, Resettlement Agency.

Priest, R., (1976). *The Homeless Person and the Psychiatric Services: An Edinburgh Survey.* British Journal of Psychiatry, 128, 128-136.

Randall, G., (1992). *Monitoring the Rough Sleepers Initiative: Report on First Audit of Rough Sleeper Sites.* Research and Information Services, London.

Randall, and Brown, (1993). *The Rough Sleepers Initiative - an Evaluation.* London, HMSO.

Reuler, J.B. and Balazs, J.R., (1991). *Portable Medical Records for Homeless Mentally Ill.* British Medical Journal, 303, 446.

Rice, J. and Donlan, P., (1992). *Housing for Health,* South East Institute of Public Health.

Rivlin, L., (1986). *A New Look at the Homeless.* Social Policy, p3-10.

Rossi, P., Wright, J., Fisher, G. and Willis, G., (1987). *The Urban Homeless: Estimating Composition and Size.* Science, 235, 1336-1341.

Roth, D. and Bean, G., (1986). *New Perspectives on Homeless Findings From a Statewide Epidemiological Study.* Hospital and Community Psychiatry, 37, 712-719.

Rowntree Trust, (1990). *Today Programme,* Radio 4, March 13.

Scheuer, M., et al, (1991). *Homelessness and the Utilisation of Acute Hospital Services in London.* King's Fund Institute, London.

Scott, J. and Boustead, M., (1991). *Characteristics of Homeless Adults in Temporary Accommodation.* British Journal of Clinical and Social Psychiatry, Supplement on Poverty.

Scott, J., (1991). *Resettlement Unit or Asylum?* Paper presented at The Royal College of Psychiatrists, Brighton, July 3.

Scott, J., (1993). *Homelessness and Mental Illness.* British Journal of Psychiatry, 162, 314-324.

Scott, R., Gaskell, P. and Morrell, D., (1966). *Patients who Reside in Common Lodging Houses.* British Medical Journal, 2, 1561-1564.

Shanks, N., (1983). *Medical Provision for the Homeless in Manchester.* Journal of the Royal College of General Practitioners, 33, 40-43.

Shelter, (1989). *Raise the Roof Campaign.* London, Shelter Publications.

Stark, C., Scott, J., Hill, M. and Morgan, W., (1989). *A Survey of the Long-Stay Users of DSS Resettlement Units, A Research Report.* London, Department of Social Security.

Stearn, J., (1987). *No Home, No Health Care?* Roof, 16-19.

Stern, R., Stilwell, B. and Henson, J., (1989). *From the Margins to the Mainstream.* London, Dramrite Printers Limited.

Stern, R. and Stilwell, B., (1989). *From the Margins to the Mainstream: Collaboration in Planning Services with Single Homeless People.* West Lambeth Health Authority, September 1989.

Stern, R., (July 1994). *Homeless People and the NHS: Are We Discriminating Enough?* Journal for Interprofessional Care.

Susser, E., Conover, M. and Struering, E., (1989). *Problems of Epidemiologic Method in Assessing the Type and Extent of Mental Illness Among Homeless Adults.* Hospital Community Psychiatry, 40, 261-265.

Susser, E., Conover, S. and Struering, E., (1990). *Mental Illness in the Homeless: Problems of Epidemiological Method in Surveys of the 1980s.* Community Mental Health Journal, 26, 387-410.

Susser, E., Struering, E. and Conover, M., (1987). *Childhood Experiences of Homeless Men.* American Journal of Psychiatry, 144, 1599-1601.

Talbott, J. and Lamb, R., (1984). *Summary and Recommendations,* p1-10. In The Homeless Mentally Ill, Ed: H. R. Lamb. Washington, American Psychiatric Association.

Tandon, P. K., (1986). *Health Care for the Homeless.* Journal of the Royal College of General Practitioners, 36, 292-294.

Thornicroft, G. and Bebbington, P., (1989). *Deinstitutionalisation - from Hospital Closure to Service Development.* British Journal of Psychiatry, 155, 739-753.

Tidmarsh, D. and Wood, S., (1972). *Psychiatric Aspects of Destitution.* In Evaluating a Community Psychiatric Service, Eds: J. Wing and A. Haley. Oxford, Oxford University Press.

Timms, P., (1990). *Psychiatric Care of the Homeless - A Domiciliary Asylum Service.* Paper presented at The Royal College of Psychiatrists Quarterly Meeting, Birmingham. July.

Tomison, A. R. and Cook, D. A. G., (1987). *Rootlessness and Mental Disorder.* British Journal of Clinical and Social Psychiatry, 5, 5-8.

Victor, C., Connelly, J., Roderick, S. and Cohen, C., (1989). *Use of Hospital Services by Homeless Families in an Inner London Health District.* British Medical Journal, 299, 725-727.

Victor, C., (1992). *Health Status of the Temporarily Homeless Population and Residents of North West Thames Region.* British Medical Journal, 305, 387-391.

Vincent, J., Trinder, P. and Unell, I., (October 1994). *Single Homelessness - Towards a Strategy for Nottingham.* Nottingham Centre for Research in Social Policy. Loughborough University of Technology.

Watson, S. and Austerberry, H., (1986). *Housing and Homelessness: A Feminist Perspective.* London, Routledge and Kegan Paul.

Weller, B., Weller, M., Coker, E. and Mohammed S., (1987). *Crisis at Christmas 1986.* Lancet, 1, 553-554.

Whiteley, J. S., (1955). *Down and Out in London: Mental Illness in Lower Social Groups.* Lancet, 2, 608-610.

Williams, R. and Morgan, H.G., (1994). *Suicide Prevention - The Challenge Confronted.* London, HMSO.

Williams, R., (1994). *Commissioning Health Services for Vulnerable People.* London, British Geriatrics Society.

Williams, R. and Richardson, G., (1995). *Together We Stand - The Commissioning, Role and Management of Child and Adolescent Mental Health Services.* London, HMSO.

Williams, S. and Allen, I., (1989). *Health Care for Single Homeless People.* London Policy Studies Institute.

Wright, J., (1987). *Selected Topics in the Health Status of America's Homeless: Special Report to the Institute of Medicine.* Massachusetts, University of Amherst.

Wright, J. D., (1987). *The National Health Care for the Homeless Programme.* In The Homeless in Contemporary Society, Eds: R. Bingham, R. Green, S. White. London, Sage.

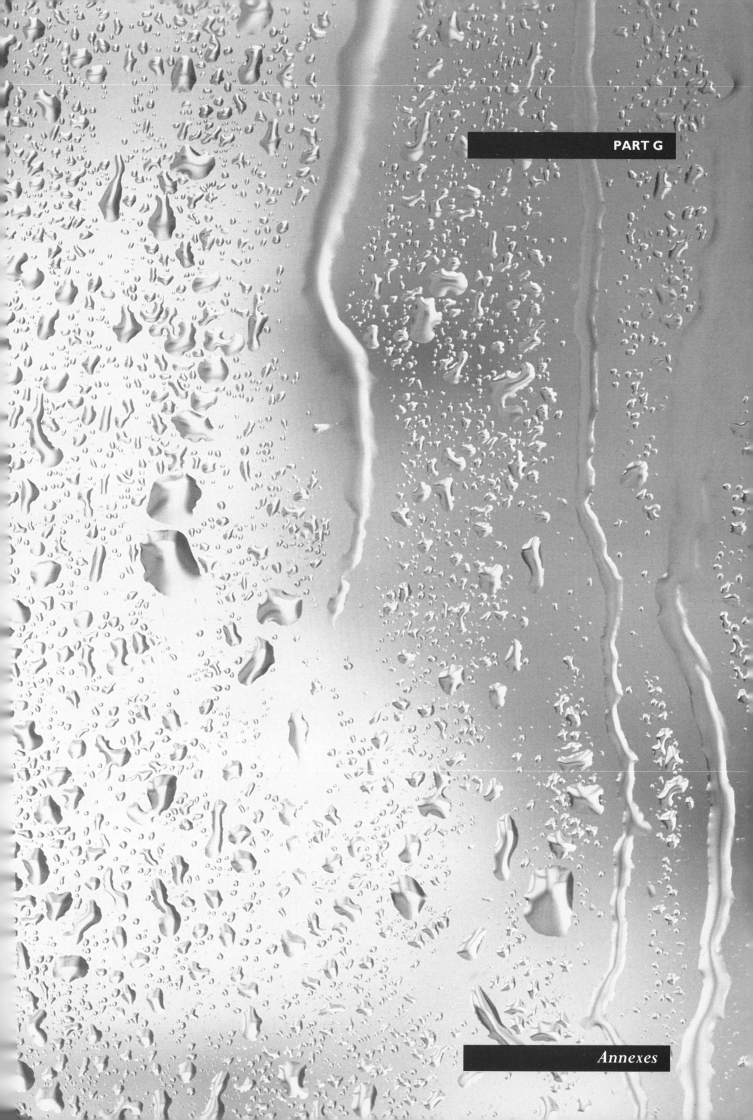

**PART G**

*Annexes*

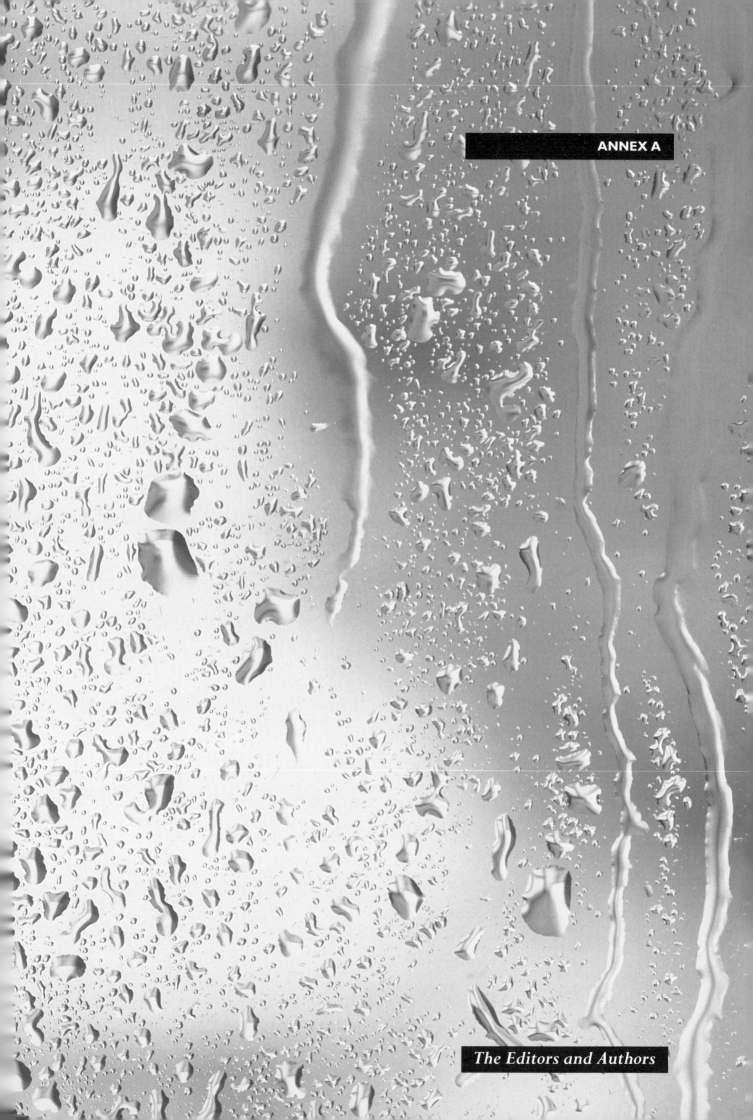

ANNEX A

*The Editors and Authors*

## Ms Kina Avebury

Ms Kina Avebury works as an independent consultant in mental health and related fields. She was previously an assistant director of MIND with responsibility for regional and community development. She subsequently worked in the Department of Psychiatry, Tower Hamlets Health Authority and latterly for the London Borough of Tower Hamlets as principal officer for mental health. She was the social services manager of the East London and the City HHELP team, which provides primary and mental health care to homeless people. She has worked extensively in the fields of homelessness, supported housing, and alcohol misuse. She is a former council member of CCETSW, co-author of *Home Life - Code of Practice for Residential Care* 1984 and a former member of a Mental Health Review Tribunal.

## Dr Simon Baugh

Dr Simon Baugh is a part-time general adult psychiatrist working at Lynfield Mount Hospital in Bradford, where he has worked as a consultant for 10 years. He has a particular interest in Community Psychiatry, working in Mental Health Resource Centres and more recently in a primary health care setting.

He is also the Director of Mental Health Services for the Bradford Community Health NHS Trust, and the Medical Director for the Trust.

## Ms Sarah Gorton

Ms Sarah Gorton has worked as the mental health worker at Health Action for Homeless People for four years. Her role is in policy and development work and aims to improve access to health and social care for single homeless people. She works with voluntary organisations, professionals from health and local authorities and policy makers. This involves raising awareness of the links between homelessness and mental distress. It seeks to identify and promote models of good practice in the delivery of health and social care which are sensitive and responsive to the needs of homeless people. Recently much of her work has been concerned with matters of community care, mental health and homelessness.

## Mr David Laws

Mr David Laws is service manager for child and adolescent mental health with the Guys and Lewisham Mental Health NHS Trust. He was previously manager of a local mental health service in East London. He is a nurse by profession and worked for five years (1988-93) in the HHELP team. In this context he was a clinical nurse specialist in mental health and homelessness, and was involved in developing the Department of Health Homeless Mentally Ill Initiative in East London. During this time, he spoke at several conferences on mental health and homelessness and joined the Royal College of Nursing's Community Mental Health Nursing Forum Executive Committee in 1991, initially to represent his specialism. He is, and has been, a member of various management committees of a number of East London voluntary organisations, many providing care to homeless people. Since 1994, he has been a member of the Advisory Group to London's Primary Care Support Force.

### Mrs Dorothy Lott

Mrs Dorothy Lott worked for six years as a group worker, counsellor and Relate counsellor before returning to college for two years. Subsequently, she worked as a social worker (ASW) in the rehabilitation and community care unit in Nottingham and has been heavily involved in the closure of two psychiatric hospitals, and in preparing people with enduring mental illness for a move into the community. After 18 months, she worked as a counselling supervisor, training and supervising telephone volunteers for Childline (Midlands). Dorothy took up her current position in 1990 as team leader of the Mental Health Support Team for Homeless People, in Nottingham. She lectures on counselling at Loughborough University's Department of Applied Social Studies, undertakes team-building for agencies throughout Nottingham City, and acts as group facilitator and supervisor to two teams in Nottingham.

### Mr Ted Riley

Mr Ted Riley is contracts manager for Avon Health Commission. He is originally from Liverpool, obtained a Business Degree from Sheffield University and worked in industry for a number of years. He subsequently trained as an occupational therapist and worked predominantly within mental health and in all arenas, including hospital and community services. Following his clinical experience, Ted moved into general management and held operational and managerial posts in occupational therapy, mental health, acute services (general surgery, operating theatres). He has also worked within a planning role in acute services.

His most recent post is with the Avon Health Commission in which he purchases and commissions services for people with mental illness, substance misuse and learning difficulties. He has also worked extensively for the NHS Health Advisory Service on several thematic reviews.

### Mr Mike Rodger

Mr Mike Rodger was a senior purchaser with the South East London Commissioning Agency after being a member of the Camberwell Health Authority district management team as general manager for the King's Dental Hospital and the Dulwich Hospital. He has had a long-standing interest in the impact of homelessness on health and was co-author of the Camberwell Health Authority 1986 strategy, *Healthcare for the Homeless*, and the joint SELCA/FHSA strategy for healthcare for homeless people, *Roots to Health*, issued in 1992. This was the first joint primary/secondary care health strategy issued in this area. He was a member of the regional steering group for the South London mental health team working with homeless people and helped to establish the South East London primary health care team for the homeless. He is now Chairman of the Nucleus Corporation, a consultancy service in the private sector.

### Professor Janine Scott

Professor Janine Scott is a professor of community psychiatry in the University of Newcastle upon Tyne. She has an interest in the psychosocial treatments of mental health problems and played a key role in the development of the Longbenton Mental Health Service which incorporates a community-based admission unit. Since 1988, she has also been involved in research on the mental health and social problems of homeless men and women. This work has particularly focused on government-run direct access hostels, and also on individuals living in temporary accommodation in provincial cities.

## Dr Richard Williams

Dr Richard Williams is the present Director of the NHS Health Advisory Service (HAS). Upon appointment in 1992, he was required to reposition the HAS so that it worked in accordance with the reformed health service. One of the new activities of the HAS, which he has developed, are the Thematic Reviews. Four of these have been completed and another seven are either close to completion or in progress. Richard Williams is also a Consultant Child and Adolescent Psychiatrist at the Bristol Royal Hospital for Sick Children, where he developed an extensive liaison and consultation service, with other community childcare workers and the child health services. His particular clinical interests include the psychological impacts and treatment of life-threatening and chronic physical disorders and he has extensive experience of working with families which have experienced psychological trauma. He has been involved in service management over a number of years and has a particular interest and experience in the theory and practice of leadership and the selection and development of leaders. Along with the Director of the Institute of Health Services Management, he inspired the creation of a Leadership Development Programme for Top Managers in Mental Health in 1994. Consequent on his work with the NHS, he has developed particular experience in the challenges posed to health authorities in purchasing comprehensive health services for mentally ill and elderly people.

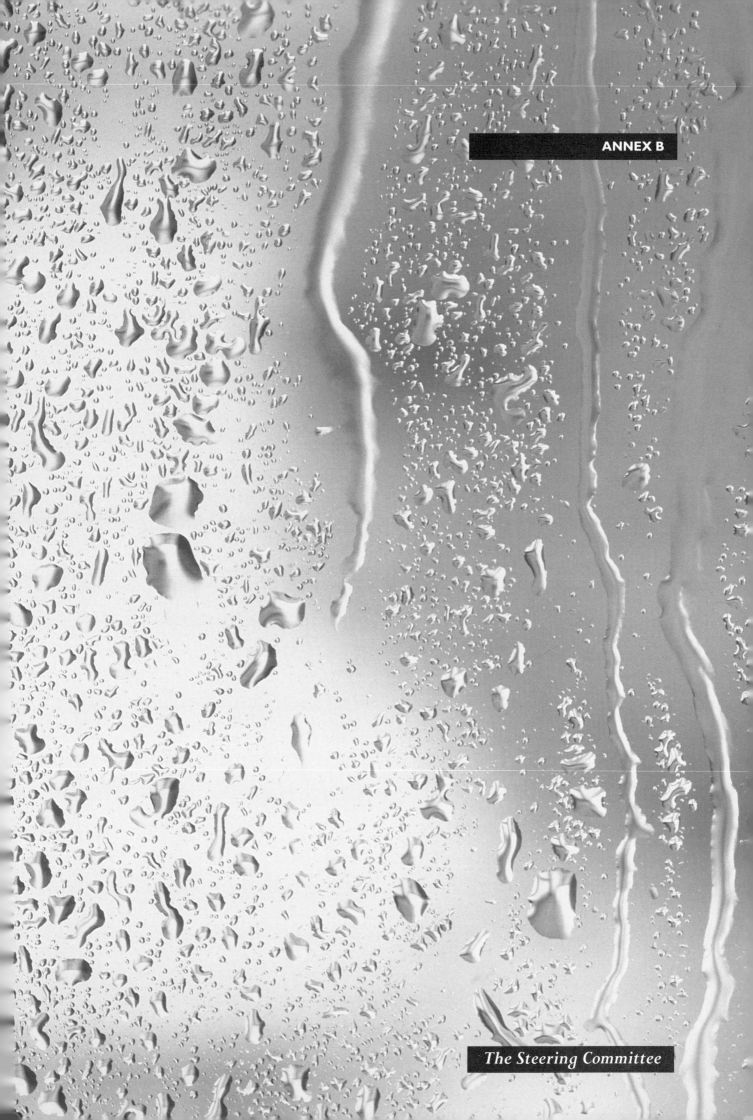

The Steering Committee

In addition to the editors and authors of this report, the steering committee for this thematic review consisted of the following:

### Dr John Balázs

Dr John Balázs is a full-time general practitioner in South London. He also works for his local purchasing health authority as an adviser on commissioning services for homeless people. He has worked with homeless people for the last eight years.

### Mr Michael G Conlon

Mr Michael Conlon was educated in Leeds and started his career in the NHS in 1959. He qualified as a nurse in 1963, and has held a number of appointments within the NHS and the independent sector. More recently, Michael Conlon has been working with the Avon Health Commission as Special Projects/Contracts Manager. During this period, he has been responsible for establishing and managing a number of primary health care projects for homeless people in the County. In addition, he has been involved in reviewing mental health services for homeless people. Furthermore, he is working with travelling people in order to assess their health care needs with them. He is also responsible for managing two needle and syringe exchange schemes, involving 22 community pharmacists and voluntary drugs' agencies. Michael Conlon is also involved in developing a pilot project to advance the care of chronic eye disease in the community.

### Dr David Cook

Dr David Cook is a senior lecturer in mental health in the University of Bristol and an honorary consultant psychiatrist to the United Bristol Healthcare NHS Trust. He has worked in the inner City of Bristol for 14 years. One of his main concerns has been with the problems of service delivery to patients in the locality, particularly in open access hostels and bed and breakfast accommodation. The community mental health team in which he works has prioritised the needs of homeless clients and clients from ethnic minorities in an effort to overcome some of the inequities of health care provision.

### Mr Ian Forster

Following training as a psychiatric nurse, Ian Forster entered social work in 1968. From 1968 to 1976 he was a student social worker, generic practitioner, fieldwork supervisor and a middle manager with four different northern local authorities.

Between 1976 and 1983, he undertook a full-time post-graduate training course, and was an adviser on mental health with North Yorkshire and Birmingham City Social Services Departments. In 1983, he joined the Internal Inspectorate of Birmingham City undertaking audit of service delivery. From 1986 to date he has been a member of the Social Services Inspectorate Wales (SSI[W]). This entails the provision of advice and support to local authorities and related agencies (through inspection, consultation and guidance), promoting good practice and assisting the Welsh Office in the formulation and promotion of policy. His policy interests have included: the All Wales Strategies for Mental Handicap and Mental Illness; HIV/AIDS; Substance Misuse; Forensic Social Work; and the works of CCETSW. SSI[W] was reorganised on 1 April 1994 and since then he has been working on a dedicated Inspection Programme with a team of full-time inspectors. He has been the SSI[W] member on an HAS review team and has represented the Welsh Office on HAS thematic review steering committees.

Ian Forster is also a member of the International Advisory Board for the Journal of Mental Health.

### Miss Mary Hancock

Miss Mary Hancock is a social services inspector in the Department of Health, with responsibility for mental health policy and mental health legislation. She is a psychiatric social worker, and has worked in Islington, Southwark and Lambeth social services departments, and as a senior lecturer in social work at Goldsmiths College. She has been involved with the Central London Homeless Mental Illness Initiative since its inception and has a long-standing interest in mental health and homelessness. She is a founder-member and past chair of London Churches Resettlement Agency, which aims to encourage church groups to produce high quality small-scale services for single homeless people.

### Mr Martin Lythgoe

Mr Martin Lythgoe's present post is that of clinical service manager, community mental health services, Guild Community Services NHS Trust in Preston. He has worked as a CPN and then a CPN manager and presently has responsibility for all community mental health services and development. Martin was, until March 1995, chair of the community mental health forum for the Royal College of Nursing contributing to mental health through a variety of channels.

### Dr Max Marshall

Dr Max Marshall is a psychiatrist and a Wellcome Health Services Research Fellow in the University of Oxford University Department of Psychiatry. His research interests include: homelessness; measuring the needs for psychiatric and social care among patients with long-term mental disorders; and assessing the effectiveness of community care.

### Ms Jan Sherlock

Ms Jan Sherlock is a psychologist who has undertaken information and development work with Good Practices in Mental Health (GPMH) for the past six years. Her first task at GPMH was to conduct a national survey of good practice in services for people with long-term mental health problems. She was involved in the Good Practices in Mental Health for Women project, and edited the resulting information pack.

The main focus of Jan's work in recent years has been raising the profile of rural mental health needs and services, by developing an information resource, regional conferences and publications. She is currently developing a rural information pack and a new information project, focusing on good practices in mental health services for young homeless people.

### Ms Tracy Stein

Ms Tracy Stein is a chartered clinical psychologist. Ms Stein worked for several years with people with long-term mental health problems in both hospital and community settings. She is a member of Access to Health, a project established by the Thames Regional Health Authorities and the King's Fund to look at services for homeless people. Tracy worked particularly in the area of mental health and primary care services for homeless people. Currently, she is working with Hillingdon Health Agency as a service development manager, commissioning a broad range of services.

## Mr Rick Stern

Mr Rick Stern is currently the commissioning development manager for South Thames RHA. Previously, he was the job-share co-ordinator of Access to Health, highlighting areas of good practice and offering support and guidance to purchasers about how to address the needs of homeless people in contracts. He was responsible for a two-year action research project in West Lambeth, reviewing the health needs of single homeless people, which led to services placing a greater emphasis on integrating homeless people into mainstream provision. He has also worked in the voluntary sector, developing supported housing services for homeless people with mental health problems. He has published a number of articles and produced a wide range of reports on the health needs of homeless people.

## Dr Phillip Timms

Dr Phil Timms is senior lecturer in community psychiatry at the Guy's and St Thomas's United Medical and Dental Schools and honorary consultant psychiatrist to the Guy's and Lewisham NHS Trust. His interest in mental illness and homelessness began during his psychiatric training at Guy's, where he conducted an epidemiological survey in a Salvation Army hostel. He helped to establish the psychiatric team for single homeless people in South London, which was the first specialist team for homeless people in the UK. Since 1991, he has been consultant psychiatrist to the multi-disciplinary mental health team, set up under the Department of Health Homeless Mentally Ill Initiative.

**ANNEX C**

*The Panel of Service Visitors*

## THE PANEL OF SERVICE VISITORS

The visits to the services were undertaken by members of the steering committee with the addition of the following professionals who were recruited for this task.

### Mrs Elizabeth Bayliss

After working with homeless women in Soho in the early 1970s, where she learnt about the failures in social policy, Elizabeth Bayliss set up a housing association which develops and manages permanent housing for homeless single people, with a range of partner agencies. She has written about primary health care and homeless people and about housing as the foundation of community care. For the last five years she has been a senior manager in the mental health services in Hackney, with a community development brief: creating several new voluntary agencies; brokering new partnerships; attracting new money; and extending the local community care infrastructure.

### Mr Roy Brooks

Roy Brooks is an independent consultant in health and social care. Qualified in social work and local government management, his social work practitioner experience was in Birmingham and the West Midlands working with older people, and with disabled and mentally ill people. He developed a managerial career in social services becoming Assistant Director, Operations, in the County of Hereford and Worcester in 1974, and three years later Deputy Director for the Metropolitan Borough of Solihull. This was followed by seven years as Deputy Director of Social Services for Northamptonshire before leaving to form his own consultancy. He has experience and expertise in organisational issues and multi-agency co-ordination with particular reference to collaboration between health and social services agencies and the work of child protection committees. His interests include housing policy, disability and mental health issues and he has well developed inspection and investigation skills.

### Dr Frank Holloway

Dr Frank Holloway is a consultant psychiatrist and the clinical director of the community directorate at the Bethlem and Maudsley NHS Trust. Formerly he was an MRC training fellow in the Academic Department of Psychological Medicine at King's College Hospital Medical and Dental School. Editor of the International Journal of Social Psychiatry. Publications and research interests focus on the evaluation of mental health services and the evolution of social policy for the mentally ill.

### Dr Susan O'Connor

Dr Susan O'Connor is a consultant psychiatrist with a special interest in elderly people. Currently she is also the clinical director of mental health services in the United Bristol Healthcare NHS Trust, Bristol. She is a Cambridge graduate and undertook her post-graduate training in Bristol. She is married with four children.

### Ms Edi O'Farrell

Ms Edi O'Farrell is currently the Director of Good Practices in Mental Health. Since qualifying as a psychiatric nurse in 1971, she has worked in a wide range of health and social services settings as a practitioner and senior manager. She has acted as a mental health consultant to health, housing and social care agencies in the UK and Europe for the past four years. She is a member of the Registered Homes Review Tribunal.

### The Panel of Service User Visitors

The following people took part in interviews with service users as part of the review:

**Brian Brecknock**

**Roberta Graley**

**Brian Hoser**

**Ian Mooney**

**Debbie Raikes**

**John Raikes**

**Steven Tyson**

**Alan Wooley**

Printed in the United Kingdom for HMSO
Dd 301189   C50   7/95   65536   3400   328560   27/33159